MRI

A Conceptual Overview

Springer

*New York
Berlin
Heidelberg
Barcelona
Budapest
Hong Kong
London
Milan
Paris
Santa Clara
Singapore
Tokyo*

Sunder S. Rajan

MRI
A Conceptual Overview

With 117 Illustrations

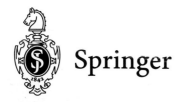

Springer

Sunder S. Rajan, Ph.D.

Library of Congress Cataloging-in-Publication Data
Rajan, Sunder S.
    MRI : a conceptual overview / Sunder S. Rajan.
        p. cm.
    Includes bibliographical references and index.
    ISBN 0-387-94911-9 (softcover : alk. paper)
    1. Magnetic resonance imaging.   2. Nuclear magnetic resonance.
I. Title
RC78.7.N83R35   1997
616.07'548—dc21   96-37408

Printed on acid-free paper.

Sunder S. Rajan, Ph.D., holds a B.Sc. (Madras Christian College), an M.Sc. (IIT Kampor), and a Ph.D. (University of Chicago), all in Chemistry. He is currently employed by Bracco Diagnostics Inc. in Princeton, NJ, as an Associate Director, Clinical Research. Prior to that, he was employed in the Department of Radiology at Georgetown University Medical Center in Washington, DC.

Production coordinated by Chernow Editorial Services, Inc., and managed by Bill Imbornoni; manufacturing supervised by Rhea Talbert.
Typeset by Best-set Typesetter Ltd., Hong Kong
Printed and bound by Maple-Vail Book Manufacturing Group, York, PA.
Printed in the United States of America.

9 8 7 6 5 4 3 2 1

ISBN 0-387-94911-9 Springer-Verlag New York Berlin Heidelberg SPIN 10559988

To my parents, Kanaka and Seshadri,
with gratitude and respect

Thanks for your patience, Sunder

Preface

Over the course of just a few decades, magnetic resonance (MR) has evolved from an analytical tool to a premier imaging modality. The ability of MR to provide cross-sectional images, as well as chemical and physiological information, has attracted students from many disciplines. Because applied MR is multidisciplinary, it is generally taught in an informal setting rather than as structured course work. During my years of teaching the subject, I felt the need for an appropriate text for students from diverse backgrounds. The materials now available are either basic introductions for the lay person or detailed reference resources providing detailed coverage of one or more aspects of MRI.

I wrote this book to supplement informal teaching with a text that will provide a detailed conceptual overview. This approach to presenting the concepts will be useful for graduate students in the physical, chemical, and biological sciences who are making the transition to MRI. In addition, medical residents, fellows, and experienced MRI technologists will benefit from this descriptive approach to MRI, which is briefly summarized in the next paragraph.

Chapter 1, an introduction to the magnetic resonance phenomenon, is followed by principles of image formation in Chapter 2. The link between the theoretical concepts introduced in Chapter 2 to the actual operation of an MRI instrument is made in Chapter 3. Chapter 4 describes the principles of image contrast, which plays a pivotal role in clinical MRI. Chapter 5, on contrast agents, introduces an exciting dimension of MRI that will continue to see progress in the coming decades. Chapter 6 provides clinical examples that will serve to inform the reader of the versatility and usefulness of clinical MRI. Chapters 7 and 8 introduce vascular imaging and spectroscopy.

MRI is rapidly progressing, and new applications continue to emerge. One of the challenges in writing this text has been to keep abreast of the rapid expansion of applications and methodology of MRI. If the book aids in providing a structured teaching tool for students of MRI despite the continuing progress in MRI technology, I will have accomplished my mission.

SURNDER S. RAJAN

Acknowledgments

This text was initially conceived as an extracurricular project with my colleagues, Drs. Mark Carvlin and Denis LeBihan, at Georgetown University. Unfortunately, they left Georgetown just after this project began. Mark was kind enough to contribute to the chapter on "Contrast Agents" and Denis to Appendix on "K-space Formalism." I would like to thank them immensely for their support, without which I would not have embarked on this long journey.

I would also like to thank my students, especially Kathleen Ward, and my friends at Georgetown, Drs. Susan Ascher, Chin-Shoou Lin, Richard Patt, Craig Platenberg, and David Thomasson, for their insights and assistance.

Thanks are also due to Alicia Montgomery for her help with the transcription and to my father-in-law Warren Grinde who was kind enough to proof the manuscript.

Last, but not least this text would have not reached completion had it not been for the constant encouragement and support of my wife, Ingrid Grinde.

Contents

Introduction to the Phenomenon of Nuclear Magnetic Resonance

Historical

Magnetic resonance imaging (MRI) has emerged as one of the most powerful diagnostic tools in the radiology clinic. The chief strengths of MRI are its ability to provide cross-sectional images of anatomical regions in any arbitrary plane and its excellent soft-tissue contrast. MRI has the ability to provide functional as well as anatomical information. The nuclear energy states of certain atoms interact with incident radio frequency photons in the presence of a static magnetic field. The radio frequency emission by tissue that follows the absorption of photons can be exploited to generate images. The phenomenon responsible for this, called the nuclear magnetic resonance (NMR) effect, was discovered almost simultaneously by Purcell and Bloch in 1946. It was recognized from the start that the nuclear magnetic resonance effect could be used to probe the electronic structure of molecules. NMR has since emerged as an invaluable analytical tool for molecular structure determination. It was only in the early 1980s that the nuclear magnetic resonance effect was exploited for imaging. In this chapter we will lay a foundation for an understanding of MRI by examining the basis of the resonance effect.

The Resonance Effect

Magnetic resonance is a phenomenon that has its origin in the magnetic properties of atomic particles such as electrons, protons, and neutrons, which form the building blocks of atoms and molecules. For reasons beyond the scope of this book, nuclei of certain atoms possess a magnetic moment. This means that they behave like a magnet, tending to align with the north pole in the manner of a compass needle. They also possess a property known as spin angular momentum, which is primarily a quantum mechanical parameter imputing to the charged nuclei an intrinsic spinning property. Both the spin angular momentum and the nuclear magnetic moment are vector quantities (i.e., they have both magnitude and direction). The behavior of a magnetic moment in the presence of an external static magnetic field is in many ways similar to that of a compass needle placed in the earth's magnetic field. Just as the compass needle tends to align itself with the north pole of the earth's magnetic field, the nuclear magnetic moment vector tends to align itself with the north pole of the static magnetic field. The presence of a spin angular momentum alters this behavior, however. The laws of physics dictate that a spinning magnetic moment will orient itself relative to static magnetic field and precess about a constant angle on the surface of a cone as shown in Figure 1.1. The most often cited analogy is that of a spinning top. The wobbly motion experienced by the top is generated by the interaction of the angular momentum of the top with the earth's gravitational field.

From the preceding section, it is evident that the preferred state (lowest energy state) of the nucleus is that of a precession at a certain angle relative to the static magnetic field. Quantum mechanics dictates that a particle with spin angular momentum will also possess a higher energy state, where the orientation is opposite to that of the first orientation. This seemingly counterintuitive property can be understood by comparing the behavior of a nuclear particle with that of a compass needle. The compass needle has a preferred energy state, which is that of alignment with the north pole. The higher energy state can be thought of as the orientation against the north pole. The number of spin energy states will depend on the spin angular momentum possessed by the nucleus. The proton, which is the simplest case, will possess two energy states (and therefore two orienta-

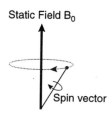

Static Field B_0

Spin vector

Figure 1.1. The orientation of a spin vector relative to the static magnetic field vector.

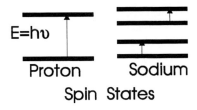

Figure 1.2. The spin energy states for proton and sodium nuclei.

tions relative to the magnetic field). On the other hand, sodium nuclei, which have a higher value of spin angular momentum, will give rise to four discrete energy states, as shown in Figure 1.2.

Given the conditions just outlined, it should be possible to detect the presence of these modified energy states by spectral excitation, as in other kinds of molecular spectroscopy. Electromagnetic radiation of the appropriate frequency should be used for spectral excitation. The appropriate frequency to be used for spin state excitation is given as follows:

$$\Delta E = h\nu \qquad (1.1)$$

Where ΔE is the difference in the energy levels, h is Planck's constant, and ν is the frequency of the photon used for excitation. When electromagnetic radiation of the correct frequency is used, resonant absorption of energy occurs. This is the underlying phenomenon exploited in magnetic resonance imaging.

An Alternate View of Resonance

The resonance effect described above may also be understood by means of an alternate approach. The applied electromagnetic radiation is an oscillating magnetic field vector (B_1), and we consider the effect on the precessing spin vectors of introducing this external oscillating field. If the frequency of the incident radiation is too high or too low compared to the precession frequency of the vector, no net response will be elicited from the precessing spin vector. This is because the relative orientations of the two vectors are constantly changing, and the spin vectors are not able to find a stable orientation (Figure 1.3, left). This situation is like two people trying to speak with each other while running laps at different speeds. When the oscillatory frequency of the B_1 vector becomes the same as that of the spin vector precession, they appear to be stationary with respect to each other. The spin vector will be affected by the B_1 vector under this condition. The spin vector will now precess relative to the B_1 magnetic field, which is the process of spin excitation (Figure 1.3,

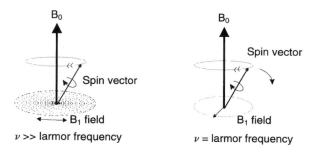

Figure 1.3. The relative positions of the spin and the B_1 vector during off-resonance and on-resonance conditions.

right). This process can be understood as a transition to a higher energy level, since the spin vector is oriented at an unfavorable angle relative to B_0.

The Larmor Equation

The separation in the spin energy levels is proportional to the magnitude of the static magnetic field and can be written as

$$\frac{\Delta E}{h} = \gamma B_0 = \nu \tag{1.2}$$

where γ is the proportionality constant and is called the gyromagnetic ratio, since the energy splitting is a manifestation of a magnetic interaction between the static field and the nuclei. The gyromagnetic ratio is a property of the nucleus, which reflects its magnetic nature. For protons, $\gamma = 42.5$ megahertz/tesla (MHz/T). Equation 1.2, which relates the resonance frequency of the photons to static magnetic field is called the Larmor equation, and the frequency ν is called the Larmor frequency. The Larmor frequencies for proton imaging at 1 and 1.5 T are 42 and 63 MHz, respectively. This falls in the radio frequency (RF) range of the electromagnetic spectrum.

Spin Ensemble Magnetization Vector

The preceding section outlined the interaction of a single spin vector with an external oscillating magnetic field. In practice, however, one is concerned with an ensemble of spins, such as in a macroscopic quantity of sample. Each of the spin vectors comprising the sample will precess at the same angle relative to the B_0 vector, although at different points on the surface of the cone (Figure 1.4).

The net effect is the vectorial sum of the spin vectors, which results in a vector parallel to the B_0 vector. (The *xy* components are random and cancel out.) This resultant spin vector arising from the macroscopic sample is termed the spin magnetization vector M_0 ($= M_z$).

At room temperature, not all spins occupy the lower energy state. In fact, only a small excess of spins occupy the lower energy level. This is because at room temperature the thermal fluctuation in energy is sufficient to cause the higher energy state to become populated. The exact ratio of the spin population is quantified by the Boltzmann equation. At progressively higher static field strengths, the lower spin energy levels are preferentially occupied. This is because of the increased value of ΔE, according to the Larmor equation. The intensity of the NMR signal is proportional to the population difference. This is because more of the spin vectors (present in the lower energy state) are available to absorb the incident RF energy. This proportionality of static field strength to NMR signal, has provided the impetus to perform MRI at progressively higher fields.

Rotating Coordinate System

In describing the spin vector dynamics during an NMR resonance, one makes use of a Cartesian coordinate system. The z-axis is arbitrarily chosen to coincide with the B_0 field vector. Let us consider the effect of the RF field vector (henceforth labeled B_1) on the spin magnetization vector M_0. In this coordinate system, the B_1 vector is shown as rotating in the xy plane, at a angular velocity v (the frequency). If v is the Larmor frequency, the magnetization vector only sees a stationary B_1 vector, since each of the spins is precessing at the Larmor frequency. This pseudostationary B_1 vector will now influence the precessing

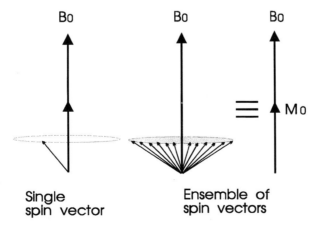

Figure 1.4. The magnetization vector generated from an ensemble of spins.

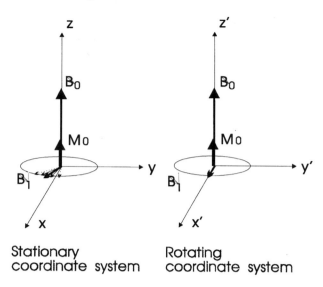

Stationary
coordinate system

Rotating
coordinate system

Figure 1.5. The B_1 vector in two frames of reference: stationary and rotating.

spins. It is therefore convenient to represent the B_1 vector as a stationary vector aligned along the x-axis, with the understanding that the entire coordinate system is rotating at the Larmor frequency. This coordinate system is represented by a primed notation (Figure 1.5).

The response of the M_0 vector to the B_1 field is a tipping motion toward the $x'y'$ plane, as though it were precessing around the B_1 field (Figure 1.6). This behavior can also be viewed as an absorption of RF energy, leading to an unfavorable orientation relative to the B_0 field. This simplified description, although adequate for the purposes of explaining most of the MRI procedures, is by no

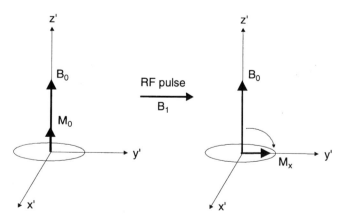

Figure 1.6. Change in orientation of the spin vector induced by the RF pulse, applied at the Larmor frequency.

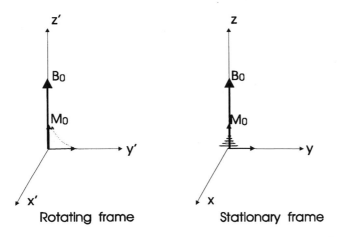

Figure 1.7. Recovery of spin magnetization in a stationary and a rotating frame of reference.

means complete. The reader is referred to more detailed treatises for a thorough understanding of the physics of spin dynamics.

The extent of tipping will depend on how long the B_1 vector is present (pulse width of the RF pulse). It will also depend on the strength of the B_1 field (voltage of the RF pulse). The angle by which the M_0 vector is displaced is an important parameter in an MR experiment and is termed the flip angle of the RF pulse. The flip angle is directly related to both the width and power of the RF pulse. Thus a 90° flip angle would place the M_0 vector along the y' axis, and a 360° flip angle would return the M_0 vector back to the z' axis. When the RF pulse is turned off, the M_0 vector will now evolve under the sole influence of the B_0 field. In the $x'y'z'$ frame, this would appear as a gradual return to the z' axis. In the xyz frame (stationary axes), however, this recovery would appear as a complex precession, as shown in Figure 1.7. The process of recovery of the spin magnetization vector, from an unstable excited state to the equilibrium value M_0, is termed **spin relaxation**.

Recovery of Magnetization (T1 and T2)

The spin relaxation properties of water protons in living tissue play a pivotal role in MRI, as we shall see in the following chapters. The actual process of spin relaxation may be vectorially decomposed into two components: the decay of the xy component and the recovery of the z component, as shown in Figure 1.8. The characteristic rate constants for the two processes are 1/T2 and 1/T1, respectively. These processes have also been termed spin–spin relaxation and spin–lattice relaxation. The

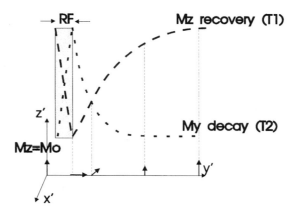

Figure 1.8. The recovery of the x and y components of the magnetization vector after the application of an RF pulse.

process of spin relaxation is inherently due to interaction of an ensemble of spin vectors with each other and cannot be explained by means of a single spin vector.

Spin–spin relaxation is caused by a gradual dispersion in the precessional frequencies, due to fluctuating local fields (from molecular motion) of the various spin vectors comprising the ensemble vector M_x. Spin–lattice relaxation is caused by thermal transfer of energy to the lattice (other molecules), thereby allowing the M_0 vector to reach a parallel orientation relative to the B_0 field. Thus it is possible for a complete decay of the M_{xy} vector (T2 decay), without a concomitant growth of the M_z vector. However, a complete recovery of the M_z vector necessitates a complete decay of the M_{xy} vector. This is another way of stating that although T1 can be longer than T2, the converse is not possible. Indeed measurements made on solid state material have found T1 to be rather long (hours) and T2 rather short (milliseconds).

The T1 and T2 relaxations are due to random molecular motion, always present at room temperature. Each spin vector is affected by the magnetic field fluctuations caused by the molecular motion of its neighbors. When the fluctuations occur in a time scale much faster than the Larmor frequency, dissipation of spin energy occurs very inefficiently. This causes T1 and T2 times to be rather long, as in liquids containing rapidly tumbling molecules (e.g., water). When the field fluctuations occur at a rate close to the Larmor frequency (e.g., protons present in lipids), exchange of energy occurs efficiently, and values for both T1 and T2 are short. If the fluctuations occur at an even slower periodicity, transfer of energy becomes inefficient; however, local field fluctuations can shorten T2 (as is seen in solid materials). It is the inherent differences in T1 and T2 relaxation times of various types of that provide the ability to discriminate NMR signal from tissue.

The oscillation of the magnetic vector during recovery, called **free precession**, causes emission of RF energy. Therefore, if a sensitive RF antenna (more precisely, a coil) is placed close to the sample, a voltage will be detected by the receiver. This voltage signal, which resembles a damped oscillation, is called a **free induction decay (FID)**. The strength of the detected FID signal is determined by the amplitude of the M_x vector. The amplitude of the M_x vector will in turn depend on the size of the M_z vector.

It is interesting to examine the effect of applying a second RF pulse before the magnetization vector has completely recovered to equilibrium value. If the M_z vector has recovered to only 50% of the equilibrium value, the M_x vector generated by the RF flip will also be only 50% of that produced the first time. Therefore, the FID signal detected is only half as strong as the first time. The size of the M_0 vector is directly proportional to the concentrations of spins. Therefore, the detected signal is also directly proportional to the concentration of the spin species.

FID and HSE Pulse Sequences

The generation of an FID from the interaction of an RF pulse and the magnetized sample is the simplest example of a pulse sequence. The pulse sequence used most often in clinical imaging is a **Hahn spin-echo (HSE)** sequence, usually referred to as a spin echo. A spin-echo sequence is constructed by adding a second RF pulse a short time (te/2) after the first RF pulse. This has an effect of forming a new signal, the **echo signal**. The echo signal is formed by the convergence of the precessing vectors, and the signal peaks at a period te/2 after the second RF pulse. The strongest echo signal is formed when the flip angles of the two RF pulses are 90 and 180°, respectively, The time period between the center of the RF pulse and the peak of the echo signal is an important parameter and is called the echo time (t_e). The FID and HSE sequences are depicted vectorially in Figure 1.9.

The formation of an HSE can be understood by examining the effect of these RF pulses on two spin vectors. In addition, the spin vectors are experiencing slightly different static fields (as is usually the case because of imperfections in the magnet). These two vectors are labeled as fast (f) and slow (s), since the vector experiencing the higher field is precessing at a faster than the other vector. The first RF pulse (90°: Figure 1.9a) flips the two vectors onto the y' axis (Figure 1.9b). During the first t_d period, the vectors diverge at a rate depending on the fields they are

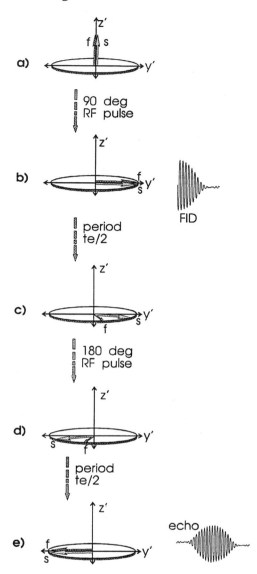

Figure 1.9. Vectorial representation of the formation of a spin echo from a 90–180° RF pulse pair.

experiencing (Figure 1.9c). The second RF pulse (180° flip) places them on the adjacent quadrant (Figure 1.9d). During the second t_d period, the two vectors are still rotating as before toward the $-y'$ axis. However, they converge at the $-y'$ axis after a time t_e, since the slower vector has a smaller arc to travel (Figure 1.9e). This act of convergence generates a peak signal from the addi-

> **Fourier Transformation** The FID waveform detected by the coil is digitized and stored in computer memory. The time domain signal is generally decomposed to its frequency components by the process of Fourier Transformation. In MRI the frequency data are ultimately used for interpretation. In imaging studies the frequency units are mapped onto spatial units, and in spectroscopy the frequency scale is used for characterization of metabolite content.

tion of the two vectors and is the echo signal. It is by means of the foregoing mechanism that a train of RF pulses will lead to the formation of a train of echo signals. The echoes cannot last indefinitely, since the T1 and T2 effects will gradually diminish the strength of the echoes.

In MRI, spin vector dynamics is exploited by tailoring specific pulse sequences using combinations of RF and magnetic field pulses. Pulse sequences can be designed to differentiate signal based on one or more spin properties (e.g., T1, T2, spin density). The chapters that follow describe the use of pulse sequences for the generation of images and for obtaining functional and biochemical information.

Additional Reading

Farrar TC, Becker ED. Pulse and Fourier transform nuclear magnetic resonance. New York: Academic Press, 1971.

Slichter CP. Principles of magnetic resonance. Springer Series in Solid-State Sciences 1. Berlin: Springer-Verlag, 1978.

2

Magnetic Field Gradient Pulses and Spatial Encoding of MR Signal

Introduction to Magnetic Field Gradient Pulses

Now that we have examined the origin of the NMR signal, we proceed to a description of the use of magnetic field gradient (MFG) pulses. Briefly, MFG pulses are utilized during an MRI scan to generate spatially encoded NMR signals, which serve in the reconstruction of an MR image. In contrast to Chapter 1, it is assumed here that the sample being exposed to the resonance effect is an object of finite size rather than a small collection of spin vectors. The static magnetic field B_0 exerted by the magnet is uniform over the entire volume of the sample. The MFG refers to an additional magnetic field applied using a separate set of current-carrying coils. The MFG is usually applied as a series of pulses during an imaging study. The direction of the MFG is along the same direction as the B_0 field (i.e., along the z axis). However, unlike the B_0 field, the field from an MFG is not uniform in the entire volume of the sample. In fact, the amplitude of the field varies linearly with distance. The amplitude can be made to vary along the x, y, or z axis independently and is generally expressed in millitesla per meter (mT/m). Figure 2.1 shows the magnetic field generated as a result of two values of MFG: 5 and 10 mT/m, along the z direction. For example, in the case of a 10 mT/m gradient pulse, the field changes by 2.5 mT at a position 25 cm from the center. It is to be noted that the gradient coils are designed to generate a symmetric change about the isocenter of the magnet.

Therefore, at a position 25 cm along the z axis, the total magnetic field during the period of the MFG pulse is $B_0 + 2.5$ mT, and it is $B_0 - 2.5$ mT at a position of -25 cm along the z direction. If the

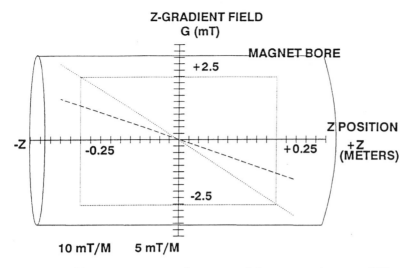

Figure 2.1. Change in B_0 as a function of distance z for two different gradient strengths.

direction of the electric current in the gradient coils is reversed, the slope of the magnetic field will be inverted. The magnetic field B_z at any point z along the z axis can be computed for a given value of gradient strength G, using the equation 2.1:

$$B_z = B_0 + (Gz) \tag{2.1}$$

The magnetic field dependence along the x and y axes can be similarly demonstrated by using separate gradient coils with suitable coil-winding geometry. Note, however, that the amplitude of the z component of the magnetic field is made to vary as a function of the x or y dimension. This point is further illustrated in Figure 2.2, which shows the magnetic field vectors when the gradient field is pulsed on in each of the Cartesian planes in a cylindrical sample.

A vector represents the magnitude and direction of the field; the length of the vector is proportional to the strength of the magnetic field. For example, the top row of Figure 2.2 shows the effect of turning on the z MFG for axial, coronal, and sagittal planes. It should be noted that all the vectors point along the z or $-z$ direction. For an arbitrary transverse plane, the field vectors are of equal length. This is because all points in this plane have the same value of z and therefore the same value of B_z according to equation 2.1. Moreover, for a given value of z, all points in the plane regardless of the x and y values will experience the same magnetic field. In the coronal and sagittal planes, the field vector varies only as a function of the $-z$ coordinate. The middle and bottom rows of Figure 2.2 depict the effect of turning on the y and x gradient fields.

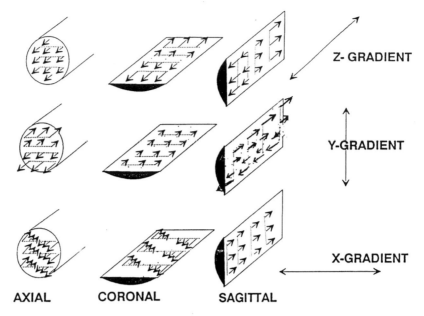

Figure 2.2. Field variation caused by gradients in the three orthogonal planes.

Radio Frequency Excitation During an MFG Pulse

Turning on a radio frequency (RF) and an MFG pulse concurrently can selectively excite a slice of the sample. Figure 2.3 shows a section across a head located at the center of a magnet. If an RF pulse at the proper frequency is turned on, all the water protons within the homogeneous region of the magnet will be excited. This result is explained by noting that all the water protons experience the same static magnetic field (B_0) and will possess the same Larmor frequency (υ_0). If a MFG pulse (z axis) is also turned on simultaneously during the RF pulse, the gradient along the z axis generates a linear distribution of Larmor frequencies.

At any given position z, the resonance frequency υ_z is given by the product of the resultant magnetic field B_z and the gyromagnetic ratio, as shown in equation 2.2.

$$\upsilon_z = \gamma B_z = \gamma(B_0 + Gz) = \upsilon_0 + \gamma Gz \qquad (2.2)$$

Table 2.1 shows the computed values of υ_z for the MFG pulse at two strengths (5 and 10 mT/m) at five points along the z axis. For all strengths of the MFG, the Larmor frequency is unaffected at the isocenter ($y = x = z = 0$). At the 12 cm position, the resonance frequency is offset by approximately 25 kHz when a gradient strength of 5 mT/m is present. If an RF pulse of a specific fre-

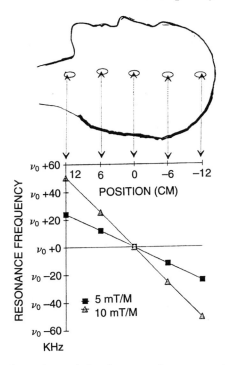

Figure 2.3. The alteration of the Larmor frequency for two different values of MFG.

Table 2.1. Some Computed Values[a] of . . .

Position (cm)	Resonant frequency (Hz)
12	63,025,200
6	63,012,600
0	63,000,000
−6	62,987,400
−12	62,974,800

[a] $\gamma = 42\,MH_z/T = 42\,keH_z/mT$
$B_0 = 1.5\,T$
Gradient $= 5\,mT/m$.

Sinc Pulses   The excitation profile of a given pulse shape is given by the Fourier transform (FT) of that pulse shape. If the shape is rectangular, the excitation profile is shaped as a sinc function ($[\sin x]/x$). Conversely, if the shape of the pulse is sinc, the excitation profile is rectangular.

rectangular   FT   sinc

quency is turned on, only spins whose resonance frequency is equal to that the frequency of the RF pulse will be affected. The magnetization vector of these spins will be tipped as described in Chapter 1. The excited spins will correspond to a transverse slice across the brain. This process of selective excitation is termed **slice selection**.

The thickness of the selected region depends on the frequency output or excitation bandwidth of the RF pulse. The bandwidth of the RF pulse is approximately equal to the inverse of the pulse width and is a complex function of the shape of the RF pulse. In practice it is necessary to excite selectively a thin slice (2–10 mm). This requires a uniform RF excitation across the slice, with minimum effect outside the thin slice (this property is referred to as a rectangular excitation profile). A sinc-shaped RF pulse (see text in box) will uniformly excite spins resonating within a narrow band of frequencies, leaving the others unaffected. For example, a bandwidth of 500 Hz can be achieved using a sinc RF pulse that is about 5 ms long. Figure 2.4 shows how two slices differing in thickness can be selected, using different values of the MFG strengths.

For example, using a gradient value of 3 mT/m allows a slice thickness of 3.9 mm. When a stronger gradient pulse (5 mT/m) is used, the precessional frequencies of the spins in this region are dispersed further. Therefore the section of the spins affected will be thinner. The slice position of the spin excitation can be chosen by tuning to the desired radio frequency. Figure 2.4 depicts an example of a sagittal slice selection. The slice selection gradient pulse and the RF pulse are first turned on. These pulses are

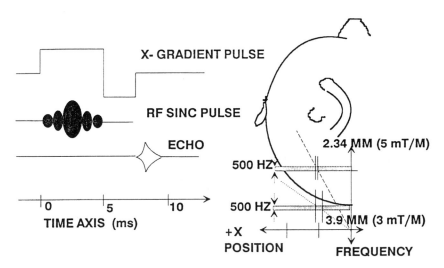

Figure 2.4. The process of slice selection and the dependence of slice thickness on gradient strength.

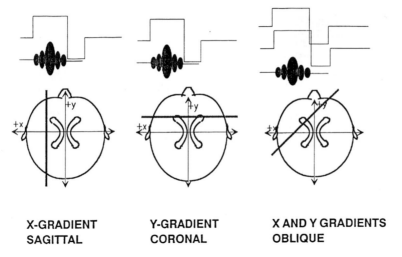

X-GRADIENT   **Y-GRADIENT**   **X AND Y GRADIENTS**
SAGITTAL   **CORONAL**   **OBLIQUE**

Figure 2.5. Selection of oblique slices by simultaneous use of two MFGs.

immediately followed by a second MFG pulse of opposite polarity. This is done to minimize intraslice signal cancellation effects due to phase dispersion. (Phase dispersion effects are further discussed in Chapter 5.) Immediately after the second MFG pulse, the FID signal generated from the slice of spins can be detected by turning on the receiver.

Slices in any orientation can be excited by choosing the appropriate gradient field according to the following tabulation:

Gradient	Plane selected
x	yz (sagittal)
y	xz (coronal)
z	xy (transverse)

Oblique slices in any arbitrary plane can also be selected by simultaneously applying two gradient pulses, as shown in Figure 2.5, where x and y gradient pulses are applied simultaneously during the slice selection period. Examination of the vectorial sums of the magnetic field vectors indicates the presence of the gradient field along the oblique direction. An extension of this reasoning can be used to understand how doubly tilted slices can be selected by simultaneously using x, y, and z gradient pulses.

Effect of Turning on an MFG Pulse During Free Precession

The behavior of the spin magnetization vectors following an RF pulse is known as free precession. A 90° flip produced by the RF

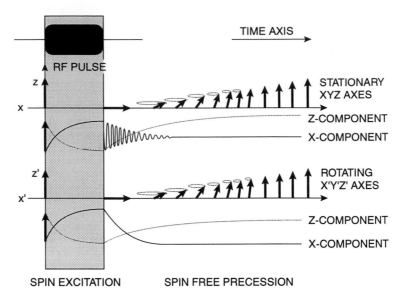

Figure 2.6. The time evolution of magnetization vectors after RF excitation in rotating (top) and stationary (bottom) coordinate systems.

pulse causes the spin magnetization vectors to align with the x' axis. After the RF pulse has been turned off, the magnetization vectors will eventually return to the z' axis. Thus the term **free precession** is used to describe the trajectory of the spin vectors during recovery toward their equilibrium state. This is best visualized vectorially using a rotating coordinate system as shown in Chapter 1 (Figure 1.5). Figure 2.6 shows free precession of the magnetization vector in a stationary (top) and in a rotating (bottom) coordinate system. In the stationary coordinate system, the magnetization vector recovers using an oscillatory motion. This is also reflected in the waveform of the x component of the vector (M_x). When the Larmor frequency is the same as that of the rotating frame, a monotonic decay of the x-magnetization is observed. If the frequencies are different, however, a damped oscillatory motion is observed. The frequency of this oscillation is equal to the difference of the Larmor and rotating frame frequencies.

To understand the effects of turning on an MFG pulse, it is essential to comprehend the concept of "phase." The relative positions of the spin vectors at any point in time during free precession comprise the **phase** of the vector. The property of phase can be attributed to any parameter that varies in a cyclic fashion, and it specifies a precise point in the oscillation. In the context of spin vector dynamics, "phase" is used to describe the relative positions of the two vectors precessing with unequal angular velocities. If two vectors start precessing at

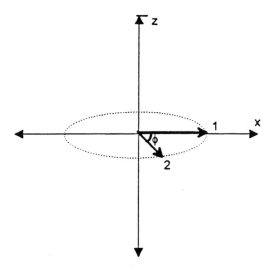

Figure 2.7. Two vectors with a phase shift of ϕ.

different points in the circle, they are said to have a phase shift relative to each other, expressed as the angle between them. Figure 2.7 shows two vectors, 1 and 2, with a phase shift of ϕ. If the vectors evolved with the same precessional frequencies, their relative phase shift ϕ will be constant. However, if for any reason the precessional frequencies are different, the phase shift will increase with time. Consider the analogy provided by the relative motions of the hour hand and the minute hand on a wall clock. Starting at 12 o'clock, the phase shift is 0. The phase shift increases to 180° as the hour and minute hand separate to 12:33, then decreases back to 0° when the clock reads 1:05.

Any mechanism that alters the Larmor frequency (e.g., the magnetic field from a gradient pulse) will cause changes in the phase of the vectors. The effect of turning on the MFG pulse during free precession in demonstrated in Figure 2.8. As before, consider the view of the brain, located in the center of the magnet.

The 90° RF pulse prepares the vectors along the x' axis of the rotating coordinating axes. The MFG pulse is turned on immediately after the RF pulse. During the MFG pulse, the precessional frequencies of the spin vectors are affected as a function of their position. On one side of the center, the spins precess faster and thereby accumulate a positive phase shift, vice versa for the other side. The total phase shift (in degrees) accumulated at any given point is a function of the distance (y value) from the center and the length of time for which the gradient pulse stays on as given in equation 2.3.

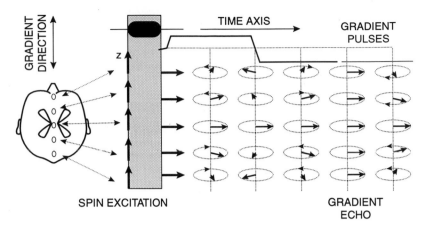

Figure 2.8. Time evolution of magnetization vectors during a gradient pulse pair, shown for five separate points along the gradient axis.

$$\Phi = \gamma G y t \times 360° \qquad (2.3)$$

where G is the gradient strength, y is the position of the spin sample, and t is the length of the gradient pulse.

The dispersion in the phases generated by the gradient pulse is reversed by the application of a subsequent gradient pulse of opposite polarity. During this period, the regions that experienced increased magnetic fields during the first MFG pulse will feel a proportionately decreased field during the second MFG, and vice versa. After a period equal to the length of the first gradient pulse, the reversal effect will be complete. At this time, the vectors from all the regions along the y axis will be realigned along the x' axis (The net phase shift is now zero). This process of realignment of the spin vectors using gradient pulses is termed a **field gradient echo**, or simply a **gradient recalled echo (GRE)**. If the gradient pulse is extended, the spin vectors will begin to diverge and will eventually dephase completely. Gradient echoes form an important class of imaging techniques, examined further in Chapters 3 and 4.

Frequency Encoding

Frequency encoding is a technique for determining the spatial origin of a gradient echo signal by virtue of its frequency. This concept is an extension of the pulse sequencing performed in Figure 2.8, whereby the receiver is used to detect echo signal formed. It was seen that during echo formation, the Larmor frequencies depend on the position of the spins along the gradient axis. Conversely, the signal detected at each frequency will arise from a unique position in the sample. The Fourier transform (FT) algorithm can be used in the observation of the frequency components of the echo signal. The intensity of the transformed signal at each frequency is proportional to the proton spin concentration at the corresponding spatial location.

To understand the effect of frequency encoding, consider a sample comprising three tubes placed 6 cm apart, in the direction of the gradient used to form the echo. Figure 2.9 demonstrates the effect of using a gradient 0.5 mT/m such that the spin will evolve at a different frequency from each of the three tubes. The Fourier transform of the echo signal will display peaks centered around the three frequencies corresponding to the distances +6, 0, −6 cm. The frequency of the signal emitted by the center tube is unaffected by the gradient pulse and is equal to the frequency of the RF pulse (e.g., 63.5 MHz). The tube placed at any given distance y will precess at a frequency given by equation 2.4:

$$\nu = \gamma B, \quad for \quad \gamma = 42.5 \text{MHz/T} \tag{2.4}$$

where $B = B_0 + B_y$, $y = 6\,\text{cm}$:

$$B_y = G_y y = \left\{ \left(0.5 \times 10^{-3}\right) \times 0.06 \right\} \text{T} = 3 \times 10^{-3}\,\text{T}$$
$$\therefore \nu = 42.5\left(B_0 + 3 \times 10^{-5}\right) = \nu_0 \text{MHz} + 1275 \text{Hz}$$

Thus the signal from the two outer tubes will occur at 2125 Hz above and below the center frequency, upon Fourier transformation. This spectral profile will resemble a projection of the cross section of the tubes, as shown in Figure 2.9. The frequency-encode procedure is also referred to as "readout," since the spatial encoding is performed while the echo signal is read out. The frequency resolution of the spectral profile will reflect the spatial resolution of the image along the readout direction. This in turn will be determined by the inverse of the data acquisition time of the echo. It is customary to use 256 or 512 data points to record the echo waveform over a period of 5 to 10 ms. The total field that is imaged is governed by the strength of the readout gradient pulse and the rate of digital recording of the echo.

Phase Encoding

Phase encoding is a technique for spatial encoding based on the phase shifts caused by a gradient pulse during free precession. As was described in Figure 2.8 and equation 2.3, an MFG pulse during free precession results in a phase shift of the vectors. The extent of the phase shift is a function of the position along the direction of the gradient pulse, the strength of the MFG pulse,

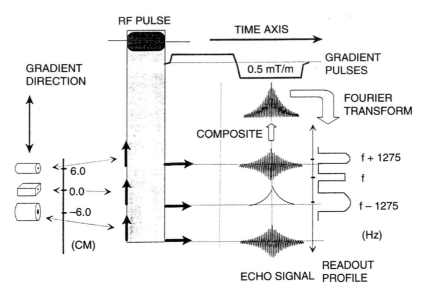

Figure 2.9. The formation of a one-dimensional profile of three sample objects by means of Fourier transformation of the frequency-encoded signal.

and the period of time during which the gradient pulse is present. Consider the phase shifts at a certain value of x (region 1) in the sample, generated from a series of experiments, each with a successively stronger gradient field as demonstrated in Figure 2.10.

The first scan shows no phase shift corresponding to zero gradient field. The second scan produces a phase shift of ϕ, from the gradient field of strength G. The third scan produces a phase shift of 2ϕ, since the gradient field is $2G$. The subsequent phase shifts are thus 3ϕ, 4ϕ. . . . If the value of ϕ is 90°, and the scan is repeated for eight steps of the gradient, ϕ will vary cyclically between 0 and 360° twice (Figure 2.10). If a different region where the ϕ is 45° is chosen (region 2), the phase shift will oscillate between 0 and 360° once. The oscillation can be thought of as a phase signal, and a frequency can be associated with it. The region with $\phi = 90$ has a phase frequency that is twice that of the region with $\phi = 45$, as is seen from the dotted curve connecting the vector tips. It is seen that every value of x has associated with it a unique value of phase frequency. It is this association that is exploited for spatial encoding of signal.

The phase frequency is found by performing a Fourier transform operation, just as in the case of frequency encoding. Using this technique, spins from various regions along the direction of the phase-encode gradient can be differentiated based on their phase frequencies. Notably, the phase frequencies can be computed after the experiment has been performed with succes-

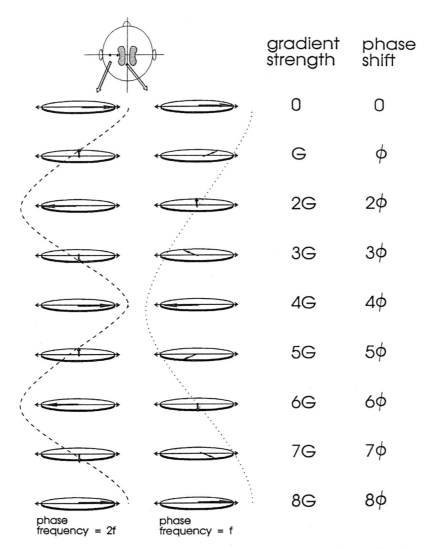

	gradient strength	phase shift
	0	0
	G	ϕ
	2G	2ϕ
	3G	3ϕ
	4G	4ϕ
	5G	5ϕ
	6G	6ϕ
	7G	7ϕ
	8G	8ϕ

phase
frequency = 2f

phase
frequency = f

Figure 2.10. The concept of phase frequency as seen from the phase shifts of two spins vectors subject to various phase-encode gradient pulses.

sively higher values of the gradient. In practice, the phase-encoded gradient is stepped from a certain negative value to a certain positive value (e.g., 256 steps). In other words, each line of frequency-encoded data is repeated 256 times, with stepped values of phase-encode gradient pulse. The recorded data for an image of a slice will consist of a matrix of points, as in Figure 2.11a. The final image (Figure 2.11c) is reconstructed by performing a Fourier transformation first along the time axis (Figure 2.11b) and then along the phase-encode direction of the data matrix. This computational algorithm, called the "2D Fourier transformation" (2DFT), is routinely used to generate MRI images. In addition, the concept of 2DFT can be readily extended to

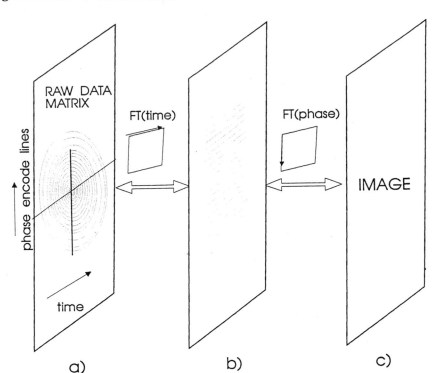

Figure 2.11. The formation of an MR image from the matrix of phase- and frequency-encoded raw data using a two-step Fourier transformation.

3D and 4D imaging. In the subsequent chapters the concepts of image generation will be further described by means of pulse sequences for dedicated applications.

Additional Reading

Mansfield P, Morris PG. In: Walsh JS, ed. NMR imaging in biomedicine. New York: Academic Press, 1982.
Stark DD, Bradley WG. Magnetic resonance imaging. 2nd ed. Chicago: Mosby-Year Book, 1992, Chapter 2.

3

MRI Hardware
System Components

Block Diagram of System Components and Overview

The MRI instrument has evolved into one of the most complex and expensive devices used in radiology practice. Advances in the instrumentation have been the single most important factor in the progress of clinical MRI. Most of this progress is due to advances in magnet and gradient coil technology, RF electronics, and computer systems.

In principle, the component requirements for an MRI instrument are quite simple. As described in Chapter 1, the hardware comprises a magnet to generate a static magnetic field, gradient coils for spatial encoding, RF electronics for irradiation and reception, and computers for data manipulation. However, the implementation of these devices requires a host of other electronics hardware. The architecture of an MRI instrument is shown in Figure 3.1, along with the various subunits and their interrelationships. In the top part of the figure is the magnet; the patient bed is on the left. The magnet is physically isolated from the rest of the system by the radio frequency shield, a metallic cage constructed from copper or aluminum sheets designed to prevent external RF (e.g., from a radio station antenna) from entering the magnet bore. Without the RF shield, the MRI coil will pick up the spurious radiation and present artifacts in the MRI images. The gradient, shim, and RF body coils are located in the center of the magnet bore. The other components (lower half of Figure 3.1) include the RF receive and transmit units, pulse sequence control units, gradient power supplies, computer console, and film output devices. Their function and operation are described later in this chapter.

Magnet

The magnetic resonance effect requires the application of a homogeneous static magnetic field, which is generated by an elec-

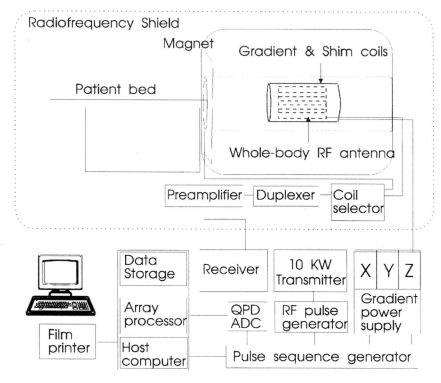

Figure 3.1. The basic components of an MR imager.

tromagnet or a permanent magnet. The magnet is constructed to allow positioning of the patient within the static magnetic field. Three types of magnet design have been available with clinical MRI systems: permanent magnets, resistive electromagnets, and superconducting electromagnets. The key features to consider in selecting a magnet design are field strength, field homogeneity, cost of maintenance, siting constraints, and patient access.

The permanent magnets are suited for low field applications, since the highest field strength achieved using a permanent clinical MR magnet is 0.3 T. These systems generally offer better patient access. Resistive and superconducting electromagnets are commercially available. Several field strengths, ranging from 0.1 T to 2.0 T, have been employed. The highest field strength approved by the US. Food and Drug Administration for clinical use is 2.0 T. In recent years, special-purpose MRI systems have become available. Figure 3.2 shows a 0.2 T magnet; its C-arm superconductive magnet design (Siemens Medical Systems) has potential for MR fluoroscopy applications.

The main difference between resistive and superconductive magnets lies in the type of material used as the electric current conductor. In the resistive magnet design, the magnetic field is generated by passing electric current through a copper coil, wound on an appropriate former. The static magnetic field is regulated by means of a dedicated power supply.

On the other hand, a solenoid winding of niobium–titanium alloy is used in the construction of superconducting magnets, and the static magnetic field is oriented parallel to the long axis of the solenoid. To generate the magnetic field, the conducting alloy is cooled to superconducting temperatures and maintained there, whereupon the current in the superconducting material is gradually increased by means of an appropriate power source. Once the desired field has been achieved, the external power source is switched off and leads of the coil are shorted simultaneously by means of a superconducting switch. In contrast to resistive conductors, virtually no dissipation of energy occurs in the superconducting state. Therefore, the magnetic field generated is constant as long as the coil is maintained in the superconducting state. In practice, superconducting magnets are very stable, with a slight monotonic loss of field over time. Resistive magnets are generally less stable and more prone to external interference.

To maintain superconductivity, the coil must be sufficiently cooled. The conductor is maintained at 8 degrees kelvin (8 K) by

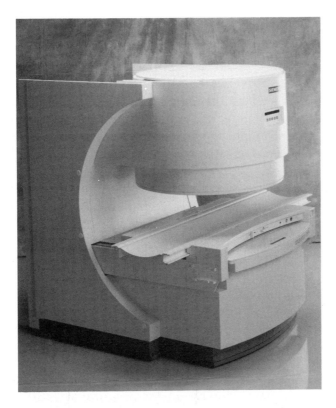

Figure 3.2. The Siemens low field MRI system MAGNETOM OPEN.

submerging it in liquid helium. To minimize losses, the liquid helium is surrounded by liquid nitrogen. The chief disadvantage with superconducting magnets is the necessity to replenish cryogen lost by evaporation. However, improved magnet construction has led to substantially lower boil-off rates of cryogen. For example, most 1.5T magnets are equipped with refrigeration units that keep the helium boil-off rates below 0.1% a day. This translates to a cryogen refill every 3–6 months. It is hoped that the development of high temperature superconducting materials will lead to the further reduction of the cryogen requirement. At this time, over 90% of the MRI magnets in use are of the superconducting type. The highest field achieved to date for whole-body imaging is 4.0T, using superconducting magnets.

An important concern is the magnetic field homogeneity afforded by the magnet. This figure of merit is generally expressed in units of parts per million (ppm) and refers to the extent to which the z component of the magnetic field varies within the bore of the magnet. To yield distortion-free images, the magnetic field should be constant to within 10 ppm. Typically, this degree of homogeneity needs to be achieved over a $50(z) \times 40(x) \times 40(y)$ cm^3 volume. For spectroscopic studies, even better homogeneity (< 0.5 ppm) is needed.

The best homogeneity that can be expected with a superconducting magnet is about 100 ppm in a 50 cm sphere. Magnetic field homogeneity is improved by the application, via auxiliary current-carrying coils, of additional fields. These coils are referred to as the **shim** coils, and by the process of iteration adjusting the shim currents to optimize the homogeneity is referred to as **shimming** the magnetic field. Alternatively, the magnetic field can be shimmed by placement of iron pieces to correct for magnetic field inhomogeneities.

The magnetic field exerted outside the magnet, referred to as the **fringe field**, is also an important parameter for siting purposes. Minimum fringe fields are desirable for reasons of keeping occupational exposure as low as possible. For a given design, the fringe fields will increase with the operating field of the magnet and with the bore size of the magnet. Also, the magnitude of the magnetic field decreases as the third power of distance from the isocenter of the magnet. The process of reducing the fringe fields is called magnetic field **shielding**.

One method of reducing fringe fields, the placement of steel plates around the magnet, has the disadvantage of adding to the weight of the magnet, necessitating the strengthening of the weight-bearing floor. Another method, called active shielding, is to null the external fields by means of suitable additional coils built into the cryostats. For any given MRI site, the extent and shape of the fringe fields must be mapped by making field mea-

---

Measurement of Field Homogeneity   Three methods can be used to estimate the homogeneity of a magnetic field. In the first method, the FID from a large spherical sample is analyzed. The Fourier transform of the FID will yield a spectral peak. The line width of the peak, expressed in ppm, will provide an estimate of the overall homogeneity. In the second method, a map of the field inhomogeneity is recorded in an imaging plane. This is done by recording the phase map of a spherical phantom, using a gradient echo sequence, for two different echo times. Subtraction of the two phase maps will generate an image, from which the field homogeneity can be computed. In the third method, a small phantom is used to measure the magnetic field repeatedly, at sample regions in space, to construct a field map. In modern magnet designs the field varies to within 5–10 ppm of the main field in a spherical region of 25 cm diameter.

---

surements. This is to ensure the isolation of regions with fringe fields in excess of 0.5 mT (5 Gauss) from the general public. A field level of <0.5 mT is considered safe for people with cardiac pacemakers, and <5.0 mT is acceptable for occupational exposure. Figure 3.3 shows field maps for a 1.5 T unshielded magnet in the xy and xz planes. The field lines are isocontours and resemble those from a magnetic dipole.

Gradient Coils

The gradient coils are used to generate spatially varying magnetic fields that are needed for imaging, as described in Chapter 2.

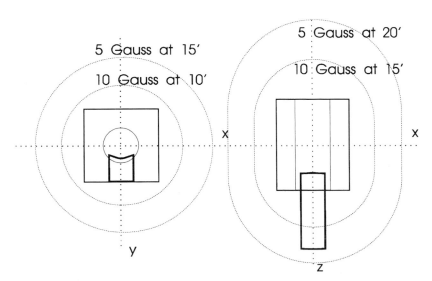

Figure 3.3. Example of fringe isocontour magnetic field lines.

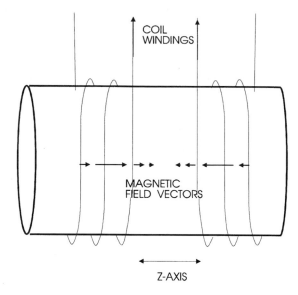

Figure 3.4. Coil windings for a z gradient.

The magnetic fields (z component) produced by the gradient coils are a linear function of distance from the isocenter of the magnet, as described in Chapter 2. The slope of this parameter is expressed as milli teslas per meter. The maximum gradient strength obtainable will ultimately dictate the spatial resolution achievable. The slice thickness achievable in multislice imaging is inversely proportional to the slice selection gradient strength. In the readout and phase-encode directions, the maximum gradient strengths will dictate the smallest field of view (FOV) attainable. A gradient strength of 10 mT/m has been found to be adequate for routine imaging of human organs and is considered a standard specification by many MR instrument vendors.

The magnetic fields for gradients are produced by passing currents through dedicated coil windings. Figure 3.4 shows how a pair of coils can be used to generate a z gradient. Since the coils are not wound in the same sense, the magnetic fields generated by passing current will be in opposite directions. This will lead to total cancellation of the field vectors between the coils, as well as progressively increasing field vectors away from the center, thus generating a gradient field. Typically, the coils are wound on a fiberglass former, which in turn is mounted inside the bore of the magnet. Once installed, the coils are rigidly mounted and are accessed infrequently (by the service engineers only). Three sets of coil windings are used, one for each of the directions x, y, and z. With such a design, the current magnitudes in each coil can be independently controlled by means of separate current amplifiers. For example, a gradient strength of about 10 mT/m will typically require a current value of about 150–200 A. For this reason, the operation of gradients will generate a considerable amount of heat and will therefore require continuous cooling.

The other major consideration in the construction of gradient coils is the **switching times** of the gradient fields: the time needed to reach maximum gradient field strength after a given coil has been energized. When the operator instructs the computer to start a pulse sequence, the sequence code is executed by the **pulse sequence generator (PSG)**. The PSG sends digital signals to the **gradient power supply** during the execution of the sequence. The digital signal is converted into an analog waveform and amplified to deliver current to the gradient coils. Two factors cause a delay in actual field pulse relative to the digital waveform driving the gradient power supply. The first is the inherent inductance of the coil, which depends on the number of coil windings. The ramp time is proportional to the inductance of the coil. The second factor is the opposing nature of the secondary induced currents in the metallic structures of the magnet. These induced currents, known as eddy currents (also called Foucault's currents), are in the opposite sense to that of the current in the coils and will cause a magnetic field that tends to cancel the field from the gradient coils (Figure 3.5). Eddy currents peak during the switching period of the gradient current and decay with characteristic times once the gradient field has reached a constant value.

The eddy current effect will therefore cause a distortion of the gradient waveform as shown in Figure 3.5. This delay can be corrected to some degree by appropriately augmenting the input current waveform. Such a modification of the input current waveform to compensate for eddy currents is called **preemphasis**. In this approach, the current value is increased in a nonlinear fashion, to overshoot the maximum value desirable. Using preemphasis, most MRI systems are capable of achieving

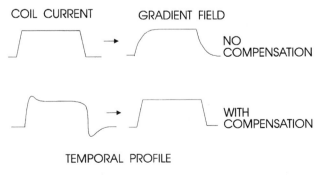

Figure 3.5. Eddy current compensation.

a 1ms ramp time for a gradient strength of 10mT/m. Alternatively, the effects of eddy currents can be minimized by constructing the gradient coils with additional windings, to minimize the gradient field in the metallic components that cause the induced currents. This active shielding approach results in higher manufacturing costs. Short switching times are of paramount importance in fast-scan MRI because of the direct dependence on the minimum echo time achievable.

Radio Frequency System Electronics

This section describes the generation of the RF pulses used in MRI. The execution of the pulse sequences requires RF irradiation of the subject, with pulses of appropriate power, frequency, phase, and pulse width, as described in Chapter 2. For example, typical spin-echo pulse sequences need narrow-bandwidth, shaped RF pulses, 1–5ms in length, for spin excitation. When the user starts the execution of a given pulse sequence, the host computer loads the appropriate timing code into the PSG. A timing code corresponding to the RF pulse is fed to the RF pulse generator, which in turn provides low voltage RF pulses of appropriate frequency and phase. The amplitude of the RF pulse can be remotely controlled by the user, for calibration of 90° and 180° flip angles, as needed in the pulse sequence.

The generation of the shaped RF pulse, described above as a single step, is actually a more complex process, which we now discuss in further detail (Figure 3.6). The shape (RF envelope) and frequency offsets (for multislice excitation) are stored in computer memory as a series of complex numbers (real and imaginary). Typically the series is composed of 256 or 512 pairs of numbers. During execution of the scan a digital-to-analog converter converts these numbers to a voltage value. This synthesizes waveform is then combined with a higher frequency

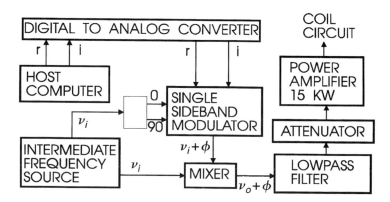

Figure 3.6. RF transmitter components.

signal, an operation that calls for the use of a single-sideband modulator to generate a waveform having a frequency equal to the sum of the two input frequencies. In some instances, the output frequency corresponds to the Larmor frequency, while in other cases it is an intermediate frequency (IF). If an IF stage is used, the frequency is further stepped up to the Larmor frequency by means of a radio frequency mixer. One of the advantages of this approach is the ease of crafting pulses for multislice selective excitations, by simply creating a text file corresponding to the real and imaginary values. The time period of the RF, hence the bandwidth, is controlled by the clock rate at which the digital complex pair is converted into an analog signal.

The low voltage RF pulse presented by the pulse generator is amplified in one or more stages by the power amplifier. The amplified output is delivered to the transmit coil by means of shielded transmission cables. The RF transmission lines are not directly connected to the coils, but are routed through a device known as a duplexer, shown previously in Figure 3.1. This duplexer isolates the sensitive receiver circuitry from the high voltage RF pulses in the transmit channel. The transmit path also includes switches that route the RF to the appropriate coils.

The receiver detects and amplifies the NMR signal generated by the spin system in response to the RF pulsing. To understand the requirements of the receiver, let us consider the nature of the NMR signal. The amplitude of the signal generated by the spin echo can vary by several order of magnitudes (10^{-5}) depending on such imaging parameters as slice thickness and in-plane resolution. Furthermore, during the course of a scan the signal level will vary from near zero to a certain maximum level for zero phase-encode gradient values. The receiver amplification must be adjustable to be able to reproduce both the low and high amplitude NMR signals. The frequency of the received signal is affected by both the slice position and the readout gradient used in the pulse sequence. The receiver system must appropriately compensate the slice-offset frequency during the course of the multislice scan, demodulating the signal by means of the same

---

Single-Sideband Modulator (SSB) The SSB performs the equivalent operation of generating the real part of the product of two complex functions. One of the complex numbers is the RF pulse waveform, and the other is the waveform of the intermediate frequency (IF). The real component of the product has a frequency equal to the sum of the IF and RF pulse waveforms and a phase equal to that of the RF pulse form.

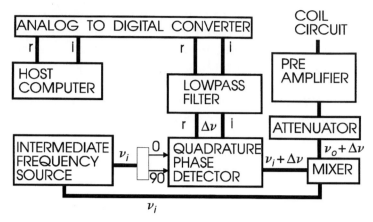

Figure 3.7. Schematic of a receiver system showing signal path.

intermediate frequency used in the transmit section. The readout gradient disperses the Larmor frequencies by about 30 kHz (Chapter 2). The image information is present in the modulated components of the carrier, within bandwidths determined by the readout gradient. These signals must be able to withstand digital sampling without loss of information when they undergo digital storage and subsequent processing. The various components of a receiver system, shown schematically in Figure 3.7, are described below.

Perhaps the most crucial component of the receiver chain is the preamplifier, which amplifies the low level signal from the coil. This is the first step in the detection process, and the most important one. The next component, designed to avoid signal overflow, is a user-controlled variable attenuator. The frequency of the signal, which is centered about the Larmor frequency, is then demodulated (stepped down) to yield components that are in the audio frequency range. This is done in much the same manner as the stepping up from RF waveform to Larmor frequency, as explained in connection with transmitters.

The audio frequencies are derived by means of a device known as the quadrature phase sensitive detector (QPD), which complements the single-sideband modulator. The carrier of audio information, along with a carrier reference, is fed into the QPD. The output of the QPD contains two channels, the real and imaginary waveforms. This method of signal detection allows recording of audio frequencies on either side of the carrier frequency. The audio waveforms (real and imaginary) are then filtered to remove high frequency noise. The use of QPD allows the bandwidth of the filters to be essentially halved in comparison to simple phase-sensitive detection. This will result in an improvement in the signal-to-noise ratio (SNR) of 1.43. Finally, an analog-to-digital converter (ADC) is used to digitize these analog wave-forms, and they are stored by the computer. The waveform is recorded during echo formation (the readout period).

The digitization of the analog signal, another crucial step in the data acquisition chain, is performed by periodic sampling of the data waveform at discrete points in time. The total length of time of data sampling will ultimately govern the frequency resolution in the readout direction. The time period between two successive samples, the dwell **time**, will determine the highest frequency sampled accurately. It is known from sampling theory that to faithfully record a periodic waveform, sampling should be done at twice the rate of the waveform. For example, to record a 1000 Hz signal accurately, one must sample the waveform at least every 500 µs. A waveform that has been sampled at two or more times its own rate is said to satisfy the Nyquist criterion for sampling, and the highest frequency waveform sampled for a given sampling rate is called the Nyquist frequency. Frequencies higher than the Nyquist frequency will be inadequately sampled and will appear as a slower waveform, as demonstrated in Figure 3.8 for the case of two frequencies (4 and the 8 Hz). The waveform is sampled at 10 Hz (data points). The waveform reconstructed by connecting the sampled points is shown below each original waveform. The reconstructed signal from 4 Hz data is accurately reproduced, but the reconstructed signal from 8 Hz data appears as a much slower (2 Hz) waveform. This misregistration phenomenon, known as frequency or Nyquist aliasing, will manifest itself as a wraparound effect in the images.

Figure 3.9 shows an example of aliasing in sagittal head image. Just as the signal frequencies that lie above the sampling limit are

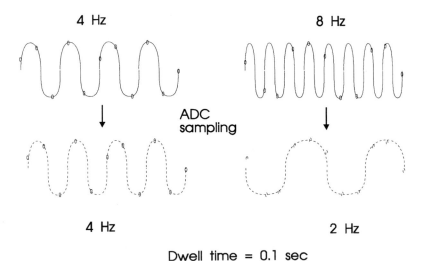

Figure 3.8. Nyquist aliasing, which results from slow sampling rates.

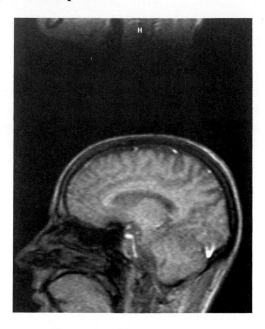

Figure 3.9. Example of frequency-encode aliasing.

subject to aliasing, so is the noise present in the receive path. Aliasing of noise will add to nonaliased noise, which can lower the signal-to-noise ratio. Low pass filters placed at the input of the ADC will minimize this effect. However, even filtering of undersampled signal often fails to completely suppress aliased signal. The only recourse is to shorten the dwell time (oversampling) so that no aliasing can occur. The unwanted higher frequency signals are then rejected after Fourier transformation, to yield an artifact-free image.

Coils and Related Electronics

The final link in the transmit–receive path to and from the patient, consists of radio frequency coils, used to efficiently transmit the RF pulses and receive the NMR signal. The coils used in magnetic resonance are resonant antennae (more precisely resonators), which are tuned to the Larmor frequency. The capacitors and inductor in the RF coil form a resonant electrical circuit. The RF current in the inductive elements of the coil generate an RF magnetic field for spin excitation; conversely, the NMR echo induces a voltage signal in the inductive elements of the coil. A simple inductor is formed by winding copper wire in the form of a solenoid. The current in the coil will generate a magnetic field within the solenoid. To ensure concentration of the magnetic field, along the x or y axis, and in the region of interest, the geometry of the inductor should be carefully chosen. In Figure

3.10, a simple example of a coil circuit, L is the inductor, Ct the capacitor (connected across the inductor that allows tuning the resonance frequency of the coil), and the capacitor Cm is used to match the impedance of the coil circuit.

The technology of coil design is an active area of interest and has seen constant progress. Most of the coils used in MRI fall into two major categories based on geometric considerations: volume coils, which provide a uniform magnetic field in the region within the coil, and surface coils, which provide a nonuniform magnetic field outside the coil. Figure 3.11 compares the field lines generated by these two coils: the shaded area corresponds to the region that can be imaged using each coil. Surface coils provide improved sensitivity at the expense of reduced image uniformity and smaller FOV.

Three types of coil design are commonly used for volume coils: the saddle, Alderman–Grant (AG), and birdcage designs. The coils used for imaging the whole body, brain, and knee typically use volume coils, which produce a magnetic field perpendicular to the long axis of the coil. The saddle coil is easier to construct but is less efficient than the other two types. The AG and bird-cage designs produce a more homogeneous magnetic field and can be modified to operate in the circularly polarized (CP) mode, in which two halves of the coil are simultaneously driven, 90 degree out of phase. Thus the vectorial sum of the two field components produces a CP magnetic field vector, used for spin excitation.

The CP field vector may be described as one whose tip re-volves around a circle of constant radius, as shown in Figure 3.12 (top). A linearly polarized (LP) vector may be described as a vector whose length oscillates between two extremes (Figure 3.12 bottom). When the coil generates an LP field during opera-tion, a CP field vector needed for spin excitation is produced by vectorial decomposition of the LP field. An LP vector can be composed by vectorial addition of two counterrotating CP vec-tors, and vice versa. Thus, if the coil generates an LP field, half the power is wasted because only one of the counterrotating components is used for spin excitation. The CP design also

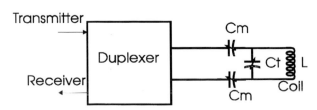

Figure 3.10. Example of a tuned coil circuit.

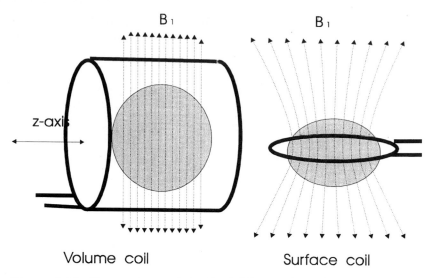

Figure 3.11. Comparison of the B_1 fields resulting from volume and from surface coils.

improves the SNR during signal reception. Most of the coils used in commercial MRI systems are of the CP type.

It has been shown that the intrinsic signal-to-noise ratio is inversely proportional to the dimension of the coil. Therefore, small coils (e.g., surface coils) for use in local imaging yield better SNRs, than the volume coils described in the preceding section. A disadvantage of using small surface coils is their inhomogenous B_1 sensitivity. The useful region of a circular surface coil extends to a hemispherical region, of radius equal to

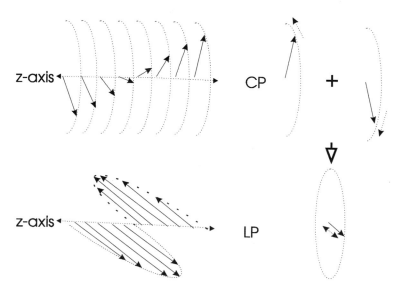

Figure 3.12. Circular and linear polarization of radiation.

Table 3.1. Coil Types and the Organs They Can Image

Coil type	Organs imaged	Notes[a]
Body	Abdomen, pelvis, cardiac	T & R, CP
Head	Brain, carotids, TMJ, ankles	T & R, CP; also used for infants
Knee	Knees, ankles	T & R, CP; also used for infants
$5 \times 10\,cm^2$ surface	Thoracic and lumbar spine, pelvis, cardiac	RO mode
Paired surface	Shoulder, TMJ wrist	T & R, RO modes; good for off-axis imaging
Neck	Cervical spine, carotids	T & R, RO modes
Array	Spine, abdomen	RO

[a]T & R, transmit–receive coil; CP, circularly polarized; RO, receive-only mode.

that of the coil. The useful region can be extended by using the surface coil for reception only, with a volume coil assigned to transmit the RF pulses. This is the scheme used in most modern MRI instruments. To be able to use two separate coils (one for transmit and the other for receiving), the coils should be mutually decoupled during operation. However, any two coils tuned to the same frequency tend to interact, and hence are difficult to decouple. The transmit and receive coils are generally decoupled by means of diode circuitry that electronically detunes one while the other is operating.

Another simple approach to coil decoupling is to mutually orient the two coils in such a way that the B_1, fields from one coil will not induce a current in the other coil. In typical operation, at least 30 dB of isolation between the two coils is necessary. If the coils are not properly decoupled, large currents are drawn by the surface coil during RF pulses. This can cause hot-spot-type artifacts in the image and can also pose a safety hazard to the subject being imaged. It is therefore stressed that these effects must be understood before a surface coil is adapted for unusual applications. Table 3.1 lists typical coil types and applications.

Additional Reading

Chen C-N, Hoult DI. Biomedical magnetic resonance technology. Medical Science Series. New York: Adam Hilger, 1989.

Fukushima E, Roeder SB. Experimental pulse NMR: A nuts and bolts approach. Reading, Mass.: Addison-Wesley Publishing Company, 1981.

4

Image Contrast and Pulse Sequences

In Chapter 2, we examined ways of applying the magnetic field gradient and radio frequency pulses to generate MRI images. The basic principles of frequency encoding, phase encoding, and slice selection were described to further an understanding of the process of image formation. The generation of an image in itself would be less useful if all types of body tissue yielded a uniformly bright image. As it turns out, the different types of tissue yield differing signal strengths based on their spin properties. This effect is responsible for the inherent image contrast arising from soft tissue for which MRI is well known. The dependence of the MR signal on spin properties can be further exploited by appropriate choice of pulse sequence and of scan parameters. The final outcome of image contrast is the result of a complex interplay of spin properties such as T1 and T2 as well as design and implementation of the pulse sequence techniques. Herein lies the versatility of the MRI technique in delineating normal anatomy as well as in characterizing pathology. In this chapter, we will study how differences in spin properties can lead to alterations in image contrast by the proper choice of pulse sequence and data acquisition parameters.

Spin Properties

The spin properties T1, T2 and spin density N are the three fundamental properties primarily responsible for generation of image contrast in tissue. The property T1 is defined as the characteristic rate of recovery of the $+z$ vector and T2 is defined as the characteristic rate of the decay of the xy components of the magnetization after the onset of an RF excitation. To date, most of the clinical MRI literature has been based on characterization of T1 and T2 contrast of normal and abnormal anatomy. More recently, other physical properties, such as flow, molecular diffusion, and chemical exchange, have been exploited for the manipulation of image contrast.

Spin Density (N)

The spin density parameter N is simply the concentration of the spins contributing to signal. In MRI, the relevant parameter is proton density $N(H)$, which refers to the proton signal. The concentration effect offers the simplest mechanism for a generation of image contrast. Thus, in the absence of T1 and T2 effects, the image intensity is primarily determined by the proton spin density $N(H)$. However, in most instances, the image signal has contributions from both lipid and water protons, which should be kept in mind. In addition, not all the water present in tissue presents an MRI signal. Only water molecules that are freely tumbling compared to bound molecules are observed. The percent of MRI-visible component can vary for the different tissue components. For example, only a weak signal (hypointense) is observed from cartilage tissue in which a relatively large number of water molecules are bound within the collagen matrix. Figure 4.1, a gradient-echo image with a ratio of pulse repetion to echo times (TR/TE) of 12/4 ms and a flip angle of 10°, displays proton density contrast. The signals from cerebrospinal fluid (CSF) and vitreous humor in the orbits are considerably brighter than the

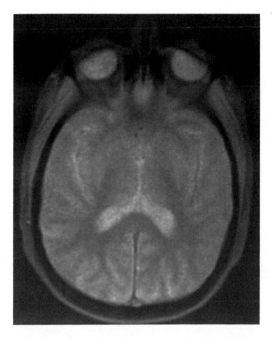

Figure 4.1. Proton density weighted image of the brain obtained using a gradient echo sequence: note bright regions corresponding to orbit and CSF.

signals from gray and white matter, which have a substantially lower proton density.

T1-Weighted Image Contrast

As described in Chapter 1, the process of RF excitation converts the equilibrium magnetization that is entirely along the +z axis to components pointing along other directions (+x,y for 90° flip, −z for 180° flip angles). The process of spin relaxation involves an exponential recovery of the +z component and a concomitant decay of the x, y components of the spin magnetization vectors. In fact, the recovery of M_{+z} occurs at the expense of the x and y components. When M_z has recovered to the equilibrium value M_0, the M_x and M_y vectors are completely dissipated. However, the converse is not always true. For example, in solid materials the T2 values are extremely short, whereas the T1 times are extremely long. This is because the dephasing of spin vectors is rather efficient and the dissipation of spin energy into the lattice is rather inefficient.

For a given RF pulse repetition time (TR), the image signal is strongly dependent on the value of T1. To understand this effect, consider two tissue components with T1 time constants of 1 and 5 seconds, respectively. The recovery of the M_0 vectors along the z axis immediately following a 90° flip RF excitation is demonstrated in Figure 4.2.

The tissue with the long TR will take 5 seconds to recover to approximately 63% of its value immediately after a 90° pulse, while the component with shorter T1 will take only 1 second. Immediately after the RF pulse, the M_z values are uniformly zero, since all the magnetization is present along the xy plane. If the FID were to be recorded at this time, the relative amplitudes of signal from both tissues would be equal. This is because the amplitude of the received signal is proportional to the M_z vector, which was flipped. Thereafter, the recovery of M_z is exponential

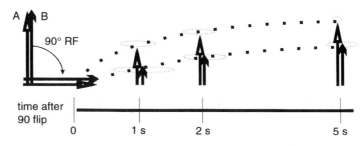

Figure 4.2. The differential T1 recovery of the M_z magnetization vectors A and B after a 90° RF excitation. The T1 times of the two components are assumed to be 1 and 5 seconds, respectively.

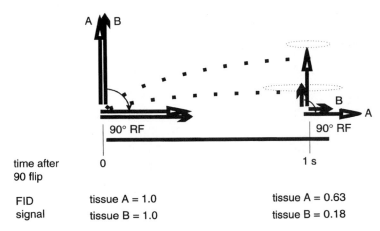

Figure 4.3. The effect of turning on a second RF pulse after a delay period of 1 second. The magnitude of the FID resulting from the second RF pulse varies inversely with the T1 values of the two species.

in time. In Figure 4.2, the size of the M_z vectors is depicted at selected points in time. The tissue with shorter $T1$ recovers to 0.63 of its original value by the first second and almost to its full original value within 5 seconds ($5 \times$ its T1 value). However, the slower relaxing tissue takes 5 seconds to reach 0.63 of its start value.

Now consider the effect of a second RF excitation (90° pulse) after an elapsed time of 1 second after the first excitation. The FID signals from the two tissue components after the second RF pulse will no longer be equal (as was the case for the first RF pulse). This is because at the time of the second RF pulse, the M_z vectors of the two recovering components were unequal. The faster relaxing spins have recovered by 0.63, whereas the spins that relax more slowly have recovered by only 0.18 of the equilibrium value. The FID signal of the two components will be approximately weighted according to the respective T1 rates, as depicted in Figure 4.3 for the two components A and B, with a T1 of 1 and 5 seconds, respectively.

We can see from the example above that the signal observed upon repeated RF pulsing is inversely related to the T1 of the tissue and increases with the TR parameter. This method of differentiating the signal from tissues with differing T1 is termed **T1 weighting**. In practice, T1 weighting is achieved by using a TR comparable to the T1 values of tissue, which lie in the range of 0.5–2.0 seconds. If a TR value that is five times larger than the T1 values is chosen, negligible T1 weighting will be observed. Figure 4.4 gives an example of changes in image signal from a two-component phantom (T1 values of 0.5 and 3 seconds, respectively) as a function of the TR parameter.

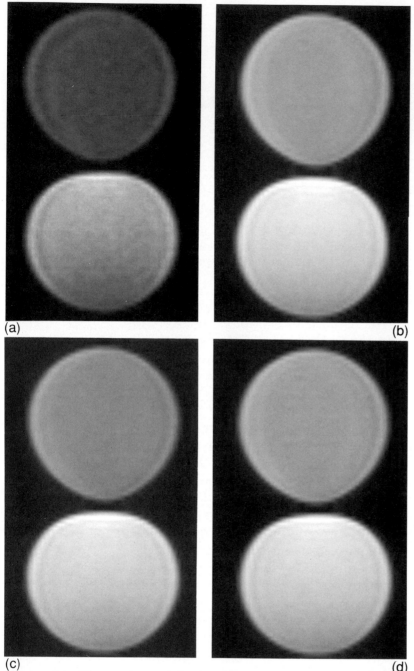

Figure 4.4. Change in signal intensity as a function of TR shown as a two-component phantom. The top phantom with short T1 shows little weighting in contrast to the bottom phantom for TR = 0.3 sec (a). As TR is lengthened, the signals are equalized, (b) 0.6 sec, (c) 1.0 sec, (d) 4.0 sec).

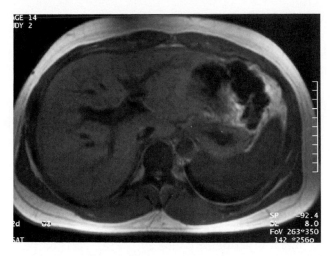

Figure 4.5. A T1-weighted gradient-echo transverse image of the body (TR/TE = 150/6 ms). The bright rim is from fatty tissue. Liver, which has a T1 shorter than muscle, is brighter than muscle. Muscle has a long T1 and thus appears relatively attenuated.

As the TR parameter is increased from 0.3 second to 4 seconds, the difference in signal between the two components decreases. The image obtained with a TR of 0.3 second displays the most T1 weighting. Changes in the contrast between any two components must always be evaluated along with changes in the overall noise. This important aspect of image contrast is discussed in the next section. Figure 4.5 is an example of a T1-weighted transverse image of the body at the level of the liver. The bright signal from fat results from the short T1 (600 ms) relative to the other components, whereas the rather long T1 (1 second) of muscle makes this tissue appear dark.

T2-Weighted Image Contrast

Just as for T1 effects, tissues with different T2 values can produce altered image intensities. This dependence of image signal on the T2 values of tissue is termed **T2 weighting**. Specifically, the decay of signal during the period between the RF excitation pulse and the acquisition of the FID (or spin echo) is responsible for differential loss of signal between the various tissue components. This T2-based loss of signal is responsible for T2-weighted image contrast and is proportional to the length of the echo time.

Consider the behavior of two tissue components with T2 values of 50 and 200 ms immediately after an RF excitation pulse. The signals from the two components recorded after a delay of 50 ms are different, as shown in Figure 4.6. During the delay period, the M_x vectors undergo exponential decay with their

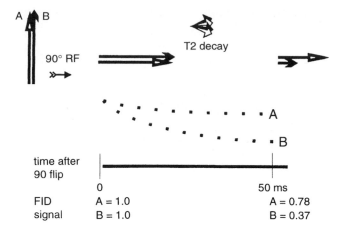

Figure 4.6. Signal loss due to T2 decay during an echo period TE of 50 ms.

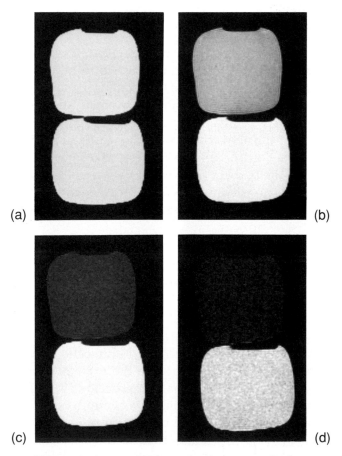

(a)

(b)

(c)

(d)

Figure 4.7. Change in image contrast as a function of echo time. (right). images of a phantom pair containing different amounts of superparamagnetic iron oxide particles (left) and transverse brain image.

respective T2 rate constants. Thus the tissue with shorter T2 presents a smaller vector (and thus a less intense image signal) than the longer T2 species. Most pulse sequences allow for a variable delay period after RF excitation during which differential T2 decay can occur and generate T2 weighting. This delay period is generally termed the **echo time (TE)**.

Figure 4.7 presents examples of T2 weighting of image contrast using a pair of phantoms containing different quantities of superparamagnetic iron oxide particles. This material has the effect of decreasing the T2 of the water protons. In addition, the T2 is inversely proportional to the concentration of the relaxation agent. The images in Figure 4.7 were acquired by means of a gradient-echo pulse sequence with varying echo times. As the echo time is lengthened from 22 ms to 135 ms, the component with shorter T2 becomes relatively less intense. Assuming that the noise value is constant, the process of T2 weighting improves the contrast between the two components.

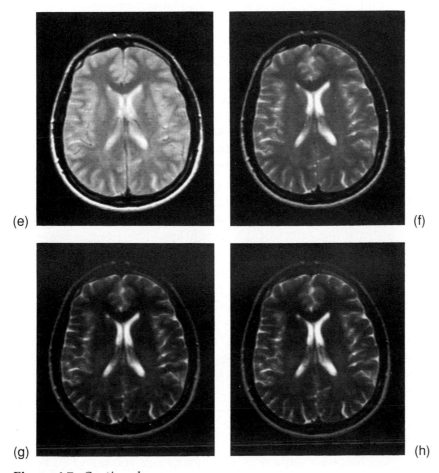

(e) (f) (g) (h)

Figure 4.7. *Continued*

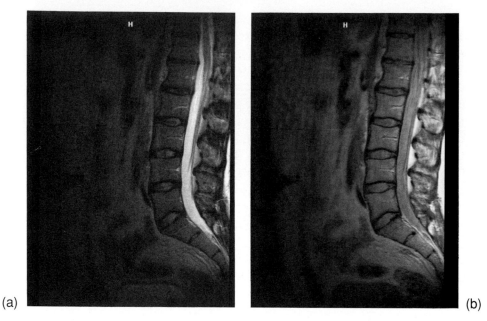

(a)   (b)

Figure 4.8. Example of T2 weighting in a sagittal lumbar image.

The images in the bottom row of Figure 4.7 demonstrate the effect of T2 weighting in the brain. At the shortest TE, minimal gray–white differentiation is noted. At longer TE values, improved contrast is noted among the tissues. As the TE is further lengthened, the overall loss of signal leads to deterioration of contrast between gray and white matter. In addition to T2 weighting, the use of rapid RF pulsing (TR comparable to T1) can produce further loss in signal by T1 weighting, as described in the preceding section. Thus T2-weighted images in practice are acquired with rather long TR values.

Figure 4.8 shows a pair of sagittal lumbar spine images to demonstrate the effect of T2 weighting. The images were acquired using a spin-echo pulse sequence, with a TR of 2500 ms and TE of 20 and 90 ms. In lengthening the TE from 20 ms to 90 ms, the relative signal from fat and cortical regions has decreased considerably, whereas the signals from CSF and brain lesions are brighter. The choice of TR in addition superimposes significant T1 weighting of the CSF, making it comparable in intensity to the surrounding spinal cord. This allows for improved visualization of white matter lesions against the gray background of the CSF.

The T2* Effect

In spin-echo pulse sequences, only processes related to T2 decay and J-coupling occur during the echo period (see Chapter 8). In gradient-echo sequences, however, B_0 nonuniformity lead to additional loss of signal. This phenomenon can be understood by examining the evolution of two vectors during a spin-echo (SE) and a gradient-echo (arc) pulse sequence. Consider two vectors labeled s and f, originating from two regions within a pixel and experiencing low and high B_0 fields, respectively. The vector f thus has a higher Larmor frequency than vector s. In the rotating coordinate frame, the echo formation is described for both an SE and a GRE sequence in Figure 4.9. For the case of SE, the refocus-

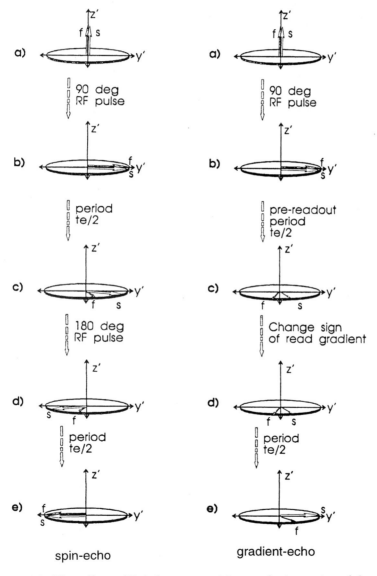

spin-echo   gradient-echo

Figure 4.9. The effect of B_0 inhomogeneities on the intensity of the echo for the case of a spin-echo (180° refocusing) pulse versus a gradient-echo (without gradient refocusing) pulse.

ing pulse places the slow vector s closer than f to the echo forma-tion axis. Thus after another echo period TE/2, the fast vector is aligned along with the slow vector during echo formation for maximum signal. When a gradient pulse is used to form an echo, the divergence of the f and s vectors is reversed as the direction of the read gradient is reversed. After a period TE/2 following gradient reversal, the vector f still retains a phase shift. This is because the gradient reversal does not fully compensate for the faster Larmor precession in the clockwise direction. This incom-plete alignment of vectors during the echo formation leads to lower image signal from that pixel. The additional B_0-induced component to the T2 relaxation in gradient-echo imaging is termed the **T2* effect**.

Diffusion Imaging

In addition to T1, T2, and proton density effects, image contrast can be altered by virtue of differences in other physiochemical properties of water in different tissues. Two such properties are the diffusion coefficient of water and the chemical exchange of water molecules. Let us briefly examine the origin of these con-trast mechanisms. The self-diffusion coefficient is a measure of the Brownian motion (random molecular motion without bulk movement) of the molecules in a liquid, and to a certain degree it is a function of size of the molecules, the local environment, and temperature. This diffusion effect is demonstrated in Figure 4.10 for a molecule that diffuses over time to cover larger and larger regions. If diffusion is completely unrestricted, the region covered by random motion is always increasing with elapsed

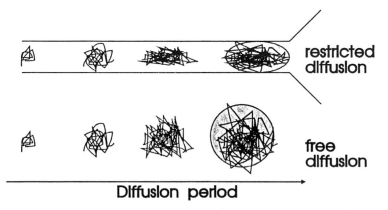

Figure 4.10. The area traversed by a molecule as a result of random motion (Brownian motion) as a function of time, for an isotropic me-dium (free diffusion) and for an anisotropic medium such as in white matter (restricted motion).

time. However, if the motion is restricted because of the local environment (cell walls, white matter tracts, etc.), the volume accessed by the random motion will level off with time. This is a caveat in the interpretation of diffusion measurements made with long diffusion times.

The diffusion coefficient represents a proportionality constant between the area traversed by molecules due to random motion with time and has units of square millimeters per second. Thus the respective diffusion coefficients of acetone and water are 4.6 $\times 10^{-3}$ and 2.2×10^{-3} mm^2/s at room temperature. Early on in the study of NMR, it was found that the strength of the spin-echo signal diminished when a field gradient pulse (e.g., a frequency-encoded gradient pulse) was turned on during the echo period. During the echo time, the spins contributing to the echo signal are undergoing phase dispersion. And, as shown in Figure 4.11, phase dispersion is increased in the presence of a gradient because of the increased range of magnetic fields (and thus increased range of Larmor frequencies) experienced by the spins as shown in Figure 4.11.

This attenuation of the spin-echo signal caused by random Brownian motion can be exploited to generate images with diffusion weighting. In biological tissue, motion can be restricted in one or more directions and can therefore yield different values of D (or diffusion weighting) based on the actual direction of the

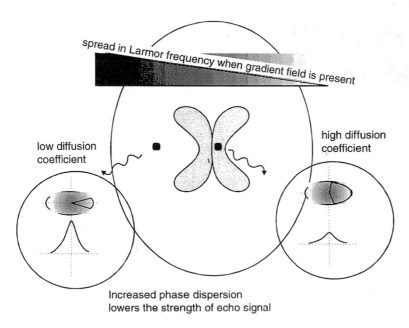

Figure 4.11. The effect of molecular diffusion on the strength of the spin-echo signal.

field gradient pulse (as is found in white matter of brain tissue). Measurements of D can be further complicated by the presence of tissue perfusion, which can artificially increase the phase dispersion and lead to overestimation of D. The brain images in Figure 4.12 were obtained with and without a diffusion gradient pulse along the anteroposterior direction. Note the pronounced

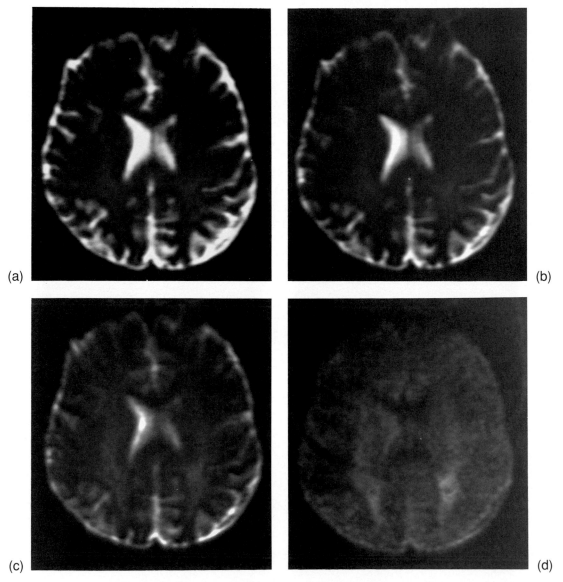

(a)

(b)

(c)

(d)

Figure 4.12. Diffusion-weighted brain images: note the pronounced attenuation of the CSF signal as a function of increasing diffusion gradient.

attenuation of CSF signal intensity due to its rather high D value, which is similar to that of free water. Performing the diffusion scan using several different values of the gradient pulse allows the computation of a diffusion image, where the gray scale represents the D value for each pixel.

The early detection of stroke presents a promising area for the application of diffusion imaging. In animal models, an ischemic insult to the brain produced within a few hours, a decrease in the D value of water in the brain tissue that could not be captured by conventional MRI techniques. The intimate connection between diffusion coefficient and temperature has led to yet another application of diffusion imaging. Diffusion imaging provides an indirect method of monitoring changes in temperature that could prove useful in hyperthermia studies. Progress in broadening the applications of diffusion imaging is currently limited by image quality problems due to the usage of strong diffusion gradients. The presence of tissue motion coupled with the use of strong gradient pulses leads to ghosting artifacts in the images, rendering the measurement of D unreliable. The availability of improved gradient hardware and faster scan methods will undoubtedly allow widespread use of this contrast mechanism.

Magnetization Transfer (MT) Contrast

Magnetization transfer (MT) provides yet another means of altering image contrast. MT refers to the coupling of magnetization of the free water protons with those of the macromolecular framework present in biological tissue. The macromolecular protons are not normally visible in a conventional image because their T2 relaxation time is extremely short (<1 ms). However, this coupling provides an additional pathway for water protons destined to undergo spin relaxation. By selectively saturating the signal from the macromolecular components, only free water spins that are chemically coupled to the saturated macromolecular components are affected. The saturation effect is transferred to the free water protons that are coupled to the macromolecular spins. This effect selectively reduces the signal of the coupled spins in the MR image. The process of saturating the macromolecular spins is carried out by using an off-resonance RF pulse as shown in Figure 4.13. An off-resonance RF pulse applied in the absence of gradients, followed by dephasing gradients, allows saturation of spins.

This approach of selectively saturating tissue signal has been exploited in imaging the blood vessels in the brain. In imaging the blood vessels, the signal from stationary tissue obscures the visualization of the blood signal. When the imaging sequence is

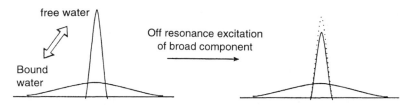

Figure 4.13. The two components of a water spectrum are connected by chemical exchange and cross-relaxation. Thus partial saturation of the broad components will be transferred to the narrow component. The reduction of signal from the free component manifests itself as decreased image intensity. Thus each line of data is preceded by an off-resonance excitation pulse.

preceded by selective irradiation of the macromolecular component of water (MTS pulse), the signal from stationary parenchymal tissue is attenuated relative to that from blood and overlying fatty tissue. This selective attenuation of the stationary signal markedly improves the conspicuity of the small blood vessels. An example of this effect is demonstrated in Figure 4.14. Note improved visualization of the smaller vessel segments in the MTS images relative to the image obtained without MTS.

Spatial Resolution and Image Contrast

Earlier sections, described the three cornerstones of MRI contrast: T1, T2, and proton density. Even if adequate contrast is present, however, the visualization of anatomical margins in MRI can be obscured by the presence of noise and poor spatial resolution. Thus, any discussion of contrast is incomplete without a consideration of spatial resolution and noise. We begin by

Fat Suppression   In imaging certain regions of the body, it is desirable to image water but suppress the fat signal. Suppression of fat signal, then, is yet another means of altering image contrast. One way to selectively suppress the fat signal is presaturation of the fat resonance just as for MTS. However, the frequency of the RF saturation pulse needs to be precisely aligned with the position (chemical shift) of the fat resonance. The presence of inhomogeneous B_0 fields further broadens the fat–water resonances, rendering the implementation of the RF saturation pulse more difficult. Since there is no chemical exchange between fat protons and the macromolecular framework, the use of an off-resonance MTS prepulse does not alter the signal intensity of fat.

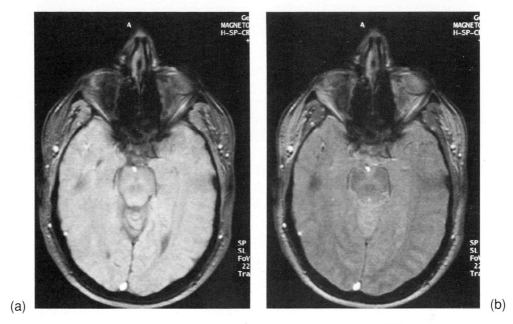

(a)   (b)

Figure 4.14. Brain MRA with (a) and without (b) MTS.

noting that the signal-to-noise ratio observed in an MRI scan is determined by two primary factors. The first relates to the inherent sensitivity of the MRI hardware, and the second comprises the volume and spin properties of the tissue that contribute to signal. The dependence of the MRI coils on SNR was discussed in Chapter 3 and is not described further. Rather, this section addresses spatial resolution and image contrast.

To understand the interrelationship between SNR and spatial resolution, let us examine what constitutes an image. An image is composed of a matrix (rows and columns) of dots and represents a slice of tissue. The intensity of each dot is proportional to the strength of the spin signal. The accuracy of this representation is directly proportional to the number of dots or, more specifically, to the density of dots per unit area. Each of the dots comprising the image is referred to as a pixel (from picture element). The accuracy of the representation is indirectly termed the "spatial resolution", in reference to the ability to resolve structures in close proximity.

In obtaining an MR image, a slice of tissue of finite thickness (1–5 mm) is first excited (refer to Chapter 2). Thus the finite thickness of the slice corresponding to the MR image will also affect the accuracy of the representation. For example, an image from a 5 mm thick slice containing a 1 mm blood vessel may completely obscure the blood vessel even if the in-plane spatial resolution is better than 0.1 mm. Thus when dealing with fine structures, it is important to extend the question about resolution to three dimensions. This admonition gives rise to the term voxel, which refers to the volume element of tissue represented by each pixel in an image. The smaller the voxel, the better the spatial resolution. On the other hand, a smaller voxel will also yield a smaller signal, since fewer protons are present in a smaller voxel than in a larger voxel. Therefore, the two most desirable attributes of an image (i.e., the SNR and spatial resolution) work against each other. In other words, as imaging parameters such as matrix size are altered to improve the resolution, the SNR is lost concurrently. In practice, diagnostic image quality is achieved through judicious choice of image spatial resolution. Any further gain in spatial resolution is offset by loss of SNR due to the smaller voxel.

In MR imaging, it is possible to vary the spatial resolution of images, at least to some degree, by changing the number of pixels comprising a given imaging field (the field of view: FOV, introduced earlier). The number of pixels in an image is determined by the number of points generated along the readout and phase-encode directions and is referred to as the matrix size of an image. This inverse relationship between spatial resolution and signal to noise is demonstrated qualitatively in Figure 4.15, using coronal section of brain images. As the matrix dimension is increased from 64×128 to 256×256, the overall image quality improves despite the drop in SNR. However, a further increase in matrix size to 256×512 does not improve the image quality, as indicated by the poor contrast between gray and white matter.

In addition to spatial resolution, contrast resolution is also a desirable attribute. **Image contrast**, the difference in signal between any two given tissue types, becomes particularly vital in determining the presence or absence of lesions. The visualization of this difference in signal (i.e., the contrast) however, is possible only if the difference in signal is significantly greater than the overriding noise (fluctuations of tissue signal). This condition has led to the use of a contrast index referred to as the contrast-to-noise ratio (CNR). The CNR is defined as the ratio of the difference in signal between any two given tissue types (S_1 and S_2) and the noise value:

$$CNR = \frac{S_1 - S_2}{noise}$$

Since the CNR directly reflects the resolving power of various tissues, it is used to evaluate the clinical efficacy of different MRI techniques toward lesion detection. Figure 4.16 shows two ex-

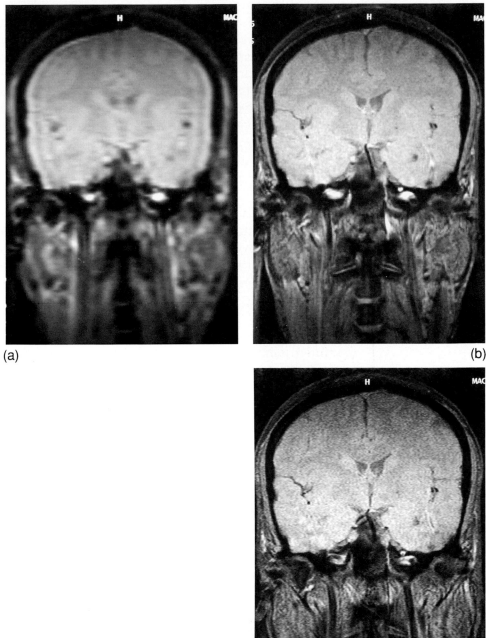

Figure 4.1.5. Coronal brain images obtained with three different matrix dimensions (diffusion gradient): (a) 0mT/m, (b) 2.5mT/m, and (c) 5mT/m.

amples of the same slice of brain tissue obtained with different CNR values: the signal from gray and white matter is attenuated on Figure 4.16b relative to Figure 4.16a. This contrast was accomplished by inserting an off-resonance magnetization transfer RF pulse, which does not alter the signal from within the blood vessel. Although the noise value between the two images is unchanged, the conspicuity of the blood vessels is markedly improved. Another commonly used example of improved contrast at the expense of SNR is seen in T2-weighted images. If the echo times are lengthened beyond a certain value, however, an overall decrease of the signal will cause a drop in the CNR.

A thorough understanding of the interrelationships between contrast, SNR, and T1 and T2 weighting is essential in the implementation of the various MRI techniques. Ultimately, every application necessitates a certain tissue contrast and a minimum spatial resolution, as dictated by the anatomical structure in question. Typical millimeter voxel dimensions are $5 \times 2 \times 2$ in body scans, $4 \times 1 \times 1$ in brain scans, and $3 \times 0.75 \times 0.75$ in orthopedic exams. These numbers are approximate and have continually improved over the years. Better detection hardware (coils) has made it possible to obtain acceptable CNR levels from smaller voxels. The contrast requirements of the scan have been attained by proper choice of pulse sequence and pulse sequence parameters, as explained in the next section.

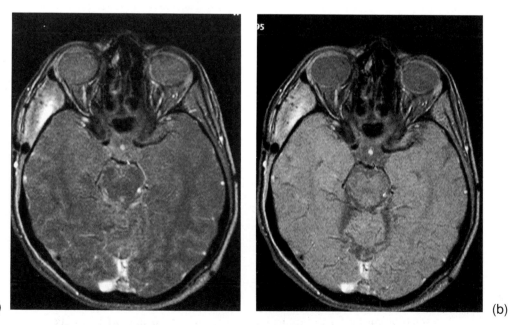

(a)   (b)

Figure 4.16. CNR of vascular signal relative to stationary tissue.

Pulse Sequences

The concept of a pulse sequence was introduced at the end of Chapter 1 in connection with the formation of a spin echo. It was further extended to image formation using a combination of radio frequency pulses and magnetic field gradient pulses (read and phasing-encoding processes). Pulse sequences thus constitute a vehicle for the generation of desirable image contrast and resolution in an MRI image. In recent years, numerous developments in MRI have led to highly specialized pulse sequences for specific clinical applications. All these pulse sequences have been derived from a few fundamental sequence types, which are described below.

In describing pulse sequences, it is customary to indicate the timing of the events corresponding to switching of RF pulses, gradient pulses, and receiver windows. Separate channels are indicated for each of the gradient channels (i.e., slice-select, read-out, and phase-encode). The simplest pulse sequence is the FID pulse sequence, which comprises a radio frequency pulse followed by an "ADC on" in the receiver channel. An imaging sequence based on the Hahn spin echo, comprising 90 and 180° RF pulses, is usually referred to as a spin-echo pulse sequence. The imaging pulse sequence that has been derived from a FID signal is the gradient recalled echo (refer to discussion of Figure 4.9). Figure 4.17 presents the schematics for an SE and a GRE sequence.

In a sequence diagram, the RF and gradient events are displayed from left to right as a function of time. For example, the pulse sequence begins with the RF pulse, which lasts approximately 2–3 ms and is displayed on the top row. The GRE sequence contains one RF pulse, whereas the spin-echo sequence contains, a 90° and a 180° RF pulse. Concurrent, with the turning on of the RF pulse is a slice-select (SS) gradient pulse, shown in the second row. This pulse is responsible for the generation of the signal from a given slice position. The slice selection process contains a positive component that occurs during the RF pulse and a negative component, which happens after the RF pulse for purposes of rephasing the spin vectors within a slice.

In the third row, the phase-encode (PE) gradient pulse is displayed as a icon for a table of gradient values. The first line of data is acquired with an extreme value of the phasing encode, and subsequent lines are acquired with step-down values until the other extreme value of the phasing code table has been reached.

The fourth row in the pulse sequence table corresponds to the readout (RO) gradient channel. For the GRE sequence, a negative

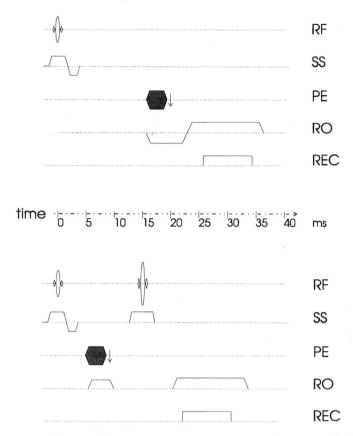

Figure 4.17. Two pulse imaging sequences: gradient recalled echo (top) and spin echo (bottom). Key: RF, radio frequency pulse; SS, slice selection; RO, readout; PE, phase-encode; REC, receiver channel on.

gradient pulse is used, followed by the refocusing of the signal to form an echo by means of a positive gradient pulse. However, for the spin echo, the first readout gradient pulse is also positive. This is because the use of a 180° refocusing RF pulse reverses the direction of the vectorial precession, which does not require gradient field reversal for echo formation.

The last row in the two pulse sequences refers to the receiver (REC) window at which the MRI signal is sampled by the receiver channel. The echo is formed when the area under the positive gradient pulse is equal to that under the first gradient pulse. The gradient magnitude and timing are adjusted to form the echo in the center of the receiver acquisition window.

As mentioned earlier, the slice selection process is repeated for every line of the phase encode gradient value, to cover the entire image (more precisely the k-space: see Appendix). In this example, the echo is formed at approximately 30ms after the RF pulse. The pulse sequence is repeated every TR period, to ensure the acquisition of the entire field of image data. Multiple slices are generally imaged during each scan, usually in an interleaved manner, as shown in Figure 4.18. For given values of TR and TE, there is a finite dead time that determines a minimum value of TR that is possible (TR_{min}). The minimum number of slices that can be imaged is given by TR/TR_{min}. In practice, many of the timing characteristics as well as the magnitudes of the gradient pulses can be altered by the user to influence the final outcome of the image.

The spin-echo pulse sequences offer an approach to generate pure T1 or T2 contrast, with minimal effect of B_0 inhomogeneity, whereas gradient-echo pulse sequences, is better suited for rapid imaging applications. In addition, the signal from flowing spins can be readily made to appear bright in GRE and dark in SE scans. The signal behavior of flowing media is considered in greater detail in Chapter 7. Most of the specialized pulse sequences used in MRI have been derived from these two basic sequence types: spin echo and GRE. Figure 4.19 shows

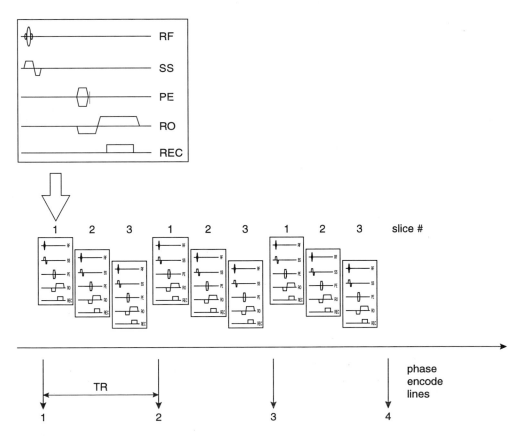

Figure 4.18. Interleaved multislice imaging.

Slice Cross Talk   When two adjacent slices of tissue are excited consecutively, slice profile imperfections may cause the region of tissue in the inner edge of the two slices to be subjected to twice the RF irradiation. This effect, known as slice cross talk, can cause signal loss. For this reason, the slice order of data acquisition is generally incremented in such a way that adjacent slice positions are not excited consecutively. The slice order used for a total of five slices is 1, 3, 5, 2, 4. In this manner the spatially adjacent slices 1, 2 are not excited consecutively.

interrelationships among the various pulse sequence techniques. On the left are techniques derived from spin echo, and on the right are techniques developed from the GRE.

The fast-spin-echo sequences (FSE) constitute an important class of pulse sequences derived from the spin echo, also called RARE, for Rapid Acquisition with Relaxation Enhancement. In this approach a train of spin echoes is generated from a single 90° RF pulse. These spin echoes are in addition subjected to increasing phase-encode gradients. Such an approach offers a significant saving in scan time. For example, a sequence that uses a

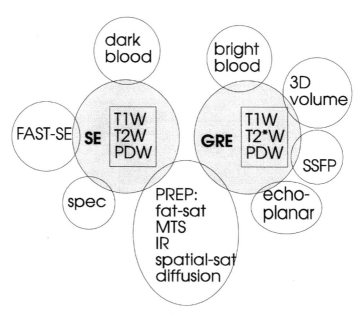

Figure 4.19. Interrelationships among the various pulse sequence methods.

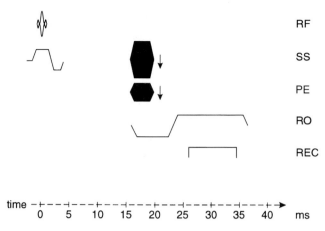

Figure 4.20. Timing diagram of a 3D-gradient-echo imaging pulse sequence; key as in Figure 4.17.

train of eight echoes offers an eightfold saving in scan time for a T2-weighted scan. However, this is not the case for a T1-weighted scan performed using a TR of 600 ms. Almost all the TR period is required to image the necessary number of slices, and any use of that precious time for more echoes will reduce the number of slices that can be acquired.

FSE sequences are routinely used instead of conventional spin-echo sequences in many applications. There is, however, an important difference in contrast behavior between the FSE and the conventional spin-echo sequences. Whereas fatty tissue appears dark in a conventional T2-weighted spin-echo image, it appears bright in an FSE image obtained with the same effective TE. Spin-echo sequences have also found use in dark-blood angiography as well as in spectroscopic imaging.

GRE sequences are useful because they allow the use of short TR values. in conjunction with small flip angles. The ability to use short TR values allows acquisition of volume data. True 3D imaging can be performed by turning on an additional set of phase-encode gradients along the slice-select channel, as shown in Figure 4.20.

GRE sequences are also commonly used to image blood flow, since the blood signal appears bright in the GRE method compared to the spin-echo method. When the TR period becomes comparable to the T2 times of the tissue in question (50–100 ms), residual x-y magnetization is still present at the start of subsequent RF excitation. Two types of sequence have evolved, based on how this residual x-y magnetization is handled. In the first type, the x-y magnetization is crushed using gradients or suitable randomization of the RF phase. These sequences are called spoiled GRE. If the residual transverse magnetization is preserved by undoing the effect of imaging gradient pulses, a steady state magnetization is produced. This is achieved by applying inverted PE, RE, and SS pulses after the echo has been recorded. Spoiled GRE sequences are useful for generating T1-weighted contrast in images. The unspoiled GRE can be designed to yield a T2* contrast in a rapid manner. However, the latter category is a special case of sequences termed steady state/free precession (SSFP) techniques.

In addition to the two basic sequences types (i.e., SE and GRE), there is another important category of sequences: here the z magnetization is prepared using a preparation RF pulse and read out using an SE or a rapid GRE sequence. Fat saturation and MTS are two common examples. Perhaps the most important preparation is the use of the inversion pulse. In this approach, all the M_z magnetization is inverted to $-M_z$ using a 180° RF pulse. Following an adjustable delay (t_i), the residual M_z magnetization is imaged. During the t_i period, T1 recovery occurs at differing rates governed by the T1s of the tissue components. Thus, for every tissue there exists a value of t_i when the signal is zero. An appropriate value of t_i can be used to selectively null one of the tissue components and improve T1 contrast. Consider an example of fat nulling in a breast image from a patient with a

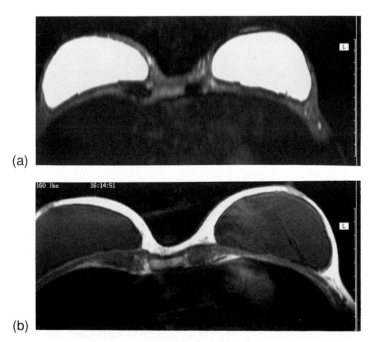

(a)

(b)

Figure 4.21. An example of fat signal attenuation using an inversion pulse. (a) with pre-inversion pulse, (b) without pre-inversion pulse.

silicone breast implant. Figure 4.21a shows fat attenuation, whereas the bright signal from fat appears in Figure 4.21b without an inversion pulse.

At present, the MRI clinician has many MRI pulse sequences available, each with certain advantages and accompanying compromises. In applications requiring reproducible T1 and T2 contrast, spin-echo sequences have been found to be most useful. In applications that must accommodate respiration, rapid GRE methods have been found to be preferable. In cardiac applications, the pulse sequences are synchronized relative to the signal of the ECG R wave. For any given choice of pulse sequence, it is generally possible to vary one or more of the scan parameters responsible for contrast. Ultimately the choice of pulse sequence and scan parameters will depend on the specifics of the diagnostic examination and the associated constraints.

Additional Reading

Edelman RR, Hesselink JR, eds. Clinical magnetic resonance imaging. Philadelphia: WB Saunders Company, 1996.

Stark DD, Bradley WG. Magnetic resonance imaging, 2nd ed. Chicago: Mosby-Year Book, 1992, Chapter 2.

gents

Magnetic resonance imaging has been recognized for its superior anatomic detail, soft-tissue contrast resolution, multiplanar capability, and noninvasive nature since the early 1980s, when it was introduced into clinical practice. These attributes have helped to establish MRI as the de facto gold standard for diagnosing most diseases of the central nervous system. Since the initial expectations of the capabilities of this technology were so high, it was felt that diagnostic pharmaceuticals to enhance image contrast would not be useful. As clinical experience using MR broadened, however, this supposition was challenged. It was found that in as many as 12% of brain tumors, the MR properties of tumor and normal brain parenchyma were sufficiently similar to allow disease to go undetected in standard T1- and T2-weighted images. The differential change in signal intensity provided by an MR contrast agent proved beneficial in resolving these ambiguities and improved the specificity of MR by highlighting regions of blood/brain barrier breakdown, by identifying the presence or absence of perfusion and/or abnormal vascularity, and by distinguishing tumor from associated edema.

MR Contrast Agent Development

The biophysical properties of tissues that contribute to magnetic resonance signal intensity and ultimately determine their appearances in the resulting MR image include the spin–lattice relaxation time (T1), the spin–spin relaxation time (T2), water content or spin density, molecular motions, flow, chemical shift, and resonant frequency. To date, modification of the spin–lattice and spin–spin relaxation times has served as the most successful basis for MR contrast agent development. As a class of compounds, chelate complexes of paramagnetic metals (Gd^{3+}, Fe^{3+}, Mn^{2+}) are effective MR contrast media because they reduce both the T1s and T2s of the hydrogen nuclei of water molecules that diffuse close to the metal ion. The relaxation times of the water molecules are altered by a magnetomolecular mechanism. The property responsible for this effect is the inherent electron paramagnetism present in the metal atom of the contrast agents. For example, Gd^{3+} and Fe^{3+} have seven and five unpaired electrons, respectively. The fluctuations of the magnetic interactions between the electron spin and proton spins provides an efficient mechanism for the dissipation of x, y, and z magnetization of the excited proton spins. This effect is a complex function of the number of unpaired electrons of the metal ion (i.e., the contrast agent), the proximity of water protons to the metal ion (i.e., the molecular structure of the ionic environment), the rate of tumbling motion of the contrast agent molecules, and the electronic spin–lattice relaxation of the metal ion. In addition to enhancing relaxation rates of the nearby water protons, the local magnetic fields can be altered, causing shifts in the resonance frequency. In practice, the paramagnetic metal ions are used as a chelated organic complex to reduce the toxicity and to tailor the magnetic property by virtue of the molecular size and structure. An example of such an agent is gadopentetate dimeglumine as shown in Figure 5.1. The ionic form of the lanthanide gadolinium is complexed to the nitrogen atoms of the ligand to form a stable chelate.

The relaxation rate of a solution containing contrast agent is a sum of the intrinsic relaxation rates (T1, T2) and contributions due to contrast agent. The latter component is proportional to the concentration of the agent. This relationship can be cast as equation 5.1:

$$\frac{1}{T_{meas}} = \frac{1}{T_0} + \frac{1}{T_{ca}}$$

$$= \frac{1}{T_0} + \left(CONC_{ca} \times R_{ca}\right) \tag{5.1}$$

where T_{meas} is the relaxation time of the contrast agent solution, T_0 is the intrinsic component (in the absence of contrast agent), and T_{ca} is the contribution due to the addition of contrast agent. The component $1/T_{ca}$ can be rewritten as a product of the concentration and R_{ca}. The parameter R_{ca}, known as relaxivity, is a property of the agent and is a measure of its ability to enhance the relaxation rates. The units of relaxivity are (millimolar $\times$ seconds)$^{-1}$ Therefore, an index of the ability of a compound to alter T1 or T2 is given by the relaxivity, R1 (for T1 effects) or R2 (for T2 effects). Figure 5.2 gives an example of T1 shortening with increasing concentrations of gadolinium complex. The effect of shortening the T1 leads to a brighter image in a T1-weighted scan, as seen in Figure 5.3.

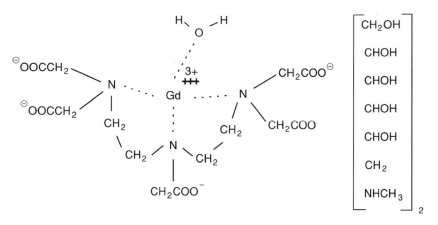

Figure 5.1. The molecular structure of a gadolinium dimeglumine agent.

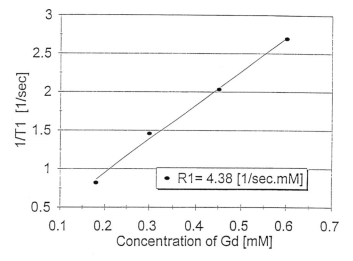

Figure 5.2. Plot T1 versus concentration of gadolinium solution. Note the linear dependence of the relaxation rate on concentration. (Courtesy of Dr. Chin-Shoou Lin.)

At present, three Gd^{3+}-based contrast agents (Magnevist, ProHance, Omniscan) have been approved by the FDA for use in clinical practice. The active ingredients (GdDTPA, GdHP-DO3A, GdDTPA-BMA) in these compounds have similar biological, chemical, and physical properties in that they are all low molecular weight chelate complexes; in addition, all distribute throughout the extracellular fluid space, all undergo renal clearance and urinary excretion, and all have comparable relaxivity values (Table 5.1).

Given the close correspondences in relaxivity, biodistribution, and pharmacokinetics among these Gd^{3+}-based agents, it is not surprising that for efficacy in a given clinical imaging application, the compounds are virtually indistinguishable. However,

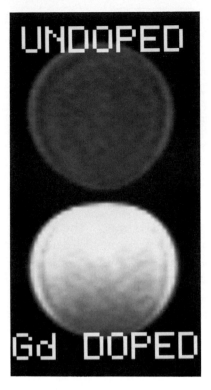

Figure 5.3. Example of increase in intensity due to T1 shortening in phantoms: images with undoped water (top) and 1 mM Gd^{3+} chelate (bottom).

these compounds are not identical in all respects. Rather, there are important differences in properties, including osmolality, viscosity, net charge, kinetic inertia to substitution of Gd^{3+} by other metal ions in vivo, and acute or chronic toxicity that may relate to drug safety (Table 5.2).

Clinical Utility of MR Contrast Media in the Central Nervous System

From the nearly 5 million contrast-enhanced MR scans performed in the world to date, distinct patterns of contrast en-

Table 5.1. Similar Properties of Gd^{3+}–Chelate MR Contrast Agents

Compound	Hydration number	Rotational correlation	Relaxivity $[(mmol \cdot s)^{-1}]$	Distribution/ $t1/2$	Elimination/ $t1/2$
Magnevist (Berlex)	1.1 ± 0.1	55	3.8 ± 0.1	Extracellular, 0.12 h	Urinary, 1.58 h
ProHance (Bracco)	1.1 ± 0.1	57	3.7 ± 0.1	Extracellular, 0.20 h	Urinary, 1.57 h
Omniscan (Nycomed)	1.1 ± 0.1	53	3.8 ± 0.1	Extracellular, 0.06 h	Urinary, 1.3 h

Table 5.2. Dissimilar Properties of Gd^{3+}–Chelate MR Contrast Agents

Compound	Lignad	Conductivity	Osmolality milliosmol/kg	Viscosity	Acid dissociation rate, K_{obs}
Magnevist (GdDTPA)	Linear, ionic	117	1960	2.9	1.2×10^{-3}
ProHance (GdDHP-DO3A)	Macrocycle, nonionic	1	630	1.3	6.3×10^{-5}
Omniscan (GdDTPA-BMA)	Linear, nonionic	5.5	650	1.4	$>2 \times 10^{-2}$

Source: Cacheris WP, Quay SC, Rockledge SM. The relationship between thermodynamics and the toxicity of gadelinium complexes. *Magn Resonance Imaging*, 8; 467–481 (1990).

hancement have been characterized, and the diagnostic value of the technique has been defined. The vast majority of clinical experiences with contrast-enhanced MR was derived from the first approved product, Magnevist, at a single recommended dose, 0.1 mmol/kg, for contrast enhancement of neurological pathology. This standard technique has proven to be very effective in demonstrating regions of abnormal vascularity and increased capillary permeability (e.g., disruption of the blood/barin barrier, as regions of increased signal intensity in postcontrast T1-weighted images. In the central nervous system (CNS), neoplastic lesions, infectious and inflammatory processes, demyelinating disease, and ischemic injury have all been evaluated using contrast-enhanced MR. The degree of contrast enhancement observed for these disease entities varies from pronounced to unremarkable and is dependent on the dose of the agent and the method by which the images are acquired, as well as the histopathologic characteristics of the target tissues.

Lesions that typically demonstrate intense enhancement using the 0.1 mmol/kg dose include meningiomas, neuromas, high grade astrocytomas, and pituitary adenomas. While the signal intensity changes are satisfactory in the majority of cases, a subset of pathologic processes exists in which enhancement may not be optimal after the administration of a dose of 0.1 mmol/kg. For agents such as Magnevist, ProHance, or Omniscan, these poorly enhancing lesions will be those that have a minimal disturbance in the blood/CNS barrier or result in only slight alterations in vascularity. In addition, the size and location of the lesion can result in poor visualization due to partial volume effects and/or insufficient contrast resolution. Brain lesions that are not consistently well visualized using standard (0.1 mmol/kg) methods include low grade astrocytoma and small/early metastatic lesions. Figure 5.4 is an example of pre- and postcontrast images of an intracranial lesion.

The variability in the degree and pattern of contrast enhancement in MR suggests that to achieve optimal visualization of

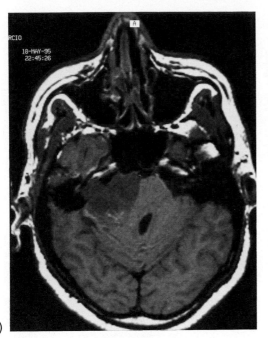 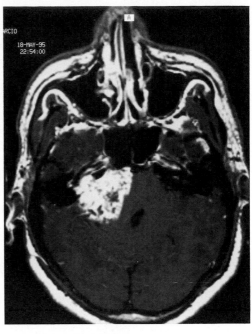

(a)

(b)

Figure 5.4. Signal enhancement of intracranial lesion upon administration of 0.1 mmol/kg of Gd^{3+} agent: (a) precontrast image and (b) postcontrast image. Note increase in the intensity of the mass in the cerebropontile angle, nasal mucosa turbinates, and blood vessels.

certain lesions, a different dose and/or a different data acquisition technique may be needed. In an early dose evaluation study conducted with Magnevist, cumulative doses greater than 0.1 mmol/kg resulted in more accurate depiction of tumorous extent as well as an increase in the number of metastatic lesions detected in a small number of patients. More recently, the hypothesis that higher doses of a Gd^{3+}-chelate contrast agent (>0.1 mmol/kg) may be indicated in certain patient populations has been put to the test in clinical trials involving each of the approved agents.

One of these studies was conducted in patients in whom the presence of cerebral metastatic disease was highly suspected. This subgroup of patients was chosen specifically because their prognosis, management, and therapy are crucially dependent on an accurate determination of the number and the location of metastatic foci. A total of 68 patients were enrolled in the study, and 48 of these were found, upon evaluation by a "blind" reader, to have radiologic evidence of metastatic disease. In 63% (30/48) of cases, the 0.3 mmol/kg dose yielded more information than was obtained from the 0.1 mmol/kg dose. This additional information pertained to an increase in the number of lesions detected

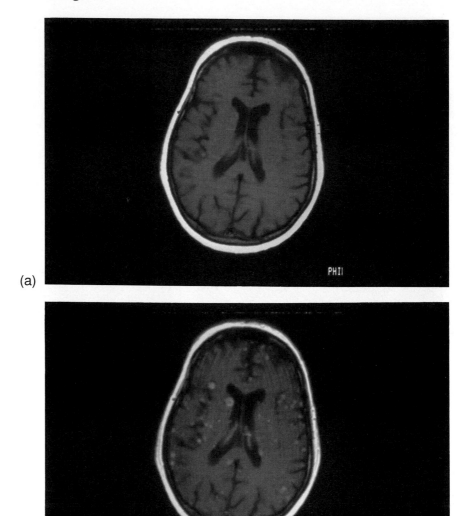

(a)

(b)

Figure 5.5. Images from the brain of a 49-year-old female refered to rale out intracraual metastases: (a) at 0.1 mmol/kg, showing no evidence of the suspected condition, and (b) at 0.3 mmol/kg, indicating extensive pathology, as described in the text. (Courtesy of Harold Friedman, MD, Northeast Illinois MRI, Prairie View, Illinois.)

in 44% (21/48) of patients. For two patients, whose 0.1 mmol/kg images showed no metastatic lesion, one metastasis was revealed in the 0.3 mmol/kg images. For five other patients, the 0.1 mmol/kg images demonstrated a solitary metastatic lesion while the 0.3 mmol/kg images showed two metastases. Comparing the 0.1 and 0.3 mmol/kg postcontrast image sets and considering all pertinent medical information for these patients, a neuro-oncologist concluded that the additional diagnostic information unique to the 0.3 mmol/kg dose over the 0.1 mmol/kg dose would have the effect of altering management and/or diagnosis in 10% (3/30) of patients. For example, a 49-year-old female was referred to rule out intracranial metastases. The larger dose revealed extensive metastatic disease that had not been detected 0.1 mmol/kg (Figure 5.5). Also detected when the larger dose was used was extensive bilateral posterior fossa cerebral metastatic involvement.

Recent dosage studies (0.1 vs. 0.3 mmol/kg) in an animal model of the postoperative spine have also shown promising results, with the higher dose providing improved differentiation of epidural scar from recurrent disk herniation. Preliminary clinical results obtained in postoperative patients show that higher doses may better delineate nerve root inflammation and epidural fibrosis after surgery on the spine.

The results of several dosing studies have indicated that doses lower than 0.1 mmol/kg are diagnostically inadequate for delineating all but selected types of CNS pathology, such as masses with a high lesion-to-background ratio on postcontrast images (acoustic neuromas) or areas with very rapid contrast uptake (pituitary adenomas, sella lesions). Also, large lesions (>10 mm), lesions associated with extensive blood/brain barrier breakdown, or lesions lacking a blood/brain barrier have been adequately visualized at doses as low as 0.025 mmol/kg.

Reduced dose applications have been identified for organ systems other than the CNS, chiefly the kidney and the heart. The rapid physiological concentration and urinary excretion of extracellular fluid space MR contrast media account for the utility of low doses in some genitourinary applications. For example, in Japan the recommended dose of Magnevist for renal imaging is 0.05 mmol/kg. Doses as low as 0.01 mmol/kg (and as high as 0.6 mmol/kg) have been employed in cardiac imaging. The extremely low dose providing contrast is informative as the acquisition parameters are adjusted to reduce the signal intensity of the myocardium and thereby make more conspicuous the distribution of the Gd^{3+}-chelate. Finally, very dilute solutions (1:250) of MR contrast media have been employed in MR arthrography for evaluation of rotator cuff tears and in the diagnosis of shoulder instability. However, practical experience with MR contrast agents at low doses is limited, and additional research is required before the appropriateness of these uses can be established. Table 5.3 summarizes criteria for indication-related dosing for Gd^{3+}-chelate MR contrast agents.

Table 5.3. Indication-Related Dosing for Gd³⁺–Chelate MR Contrast Agents

Dosing	Indications
Low ($<0.1\,$mmol/kg)	Lesions with high intrinsic contrast (L/B ratio) Tissues with physiologic concentrating ability CNS lesions with extensive blood/brain barrier disturbance CNS lesions lacking a blood/brain barrier Pituitary lesions
Standard ($0.1\,$mmol/kg)	Most CNS pathology, including: lesions associated with increased capillary permeability and lesions associated with abnormal vascularity
High ($>0.1\,$mmol/kg)	Lesions requiring higher degree of diagnostic sensitivity Lesions associated with minimal blood/brain barrier disturbance Small lesions Dynamic/functional analyses Postoperative spine

New Contrast Agents

At least a dozen new MR contrast agents are being evaluated for safety and efficacy in preliminary clinical trials. These compounds are being developed as bowel markers, hepatic/

Table 5.4. New Contrast Agents: In Clinical Trials

Agent	Application	Comments
AMI-121	Gastro intestinal	Superparamagnetic particles, T2 (dark)
OMR 12200	Grastro intestinal	Fe(III) solution, upper GI, T1 (bright)
BMS 181448	Gastro intestinal	Mn(II) solution, T1 (bright) and T2 (dark)
OMP	Gastro intestinal	Superparamagnetic particles, T2 (dark)
GdDO3A-butriol	Extracellular fluid	New generation Gd³⁺–chelate, macrocyclic and nonionic ligand
MnDPDP	Hepatobiliary	Liver, spleen, pancreas, T1 (bright)
GdBOPTA	Hepatobiliary	Liver, brain, heart, T1 (bright)
AMI-25	Hepatobiliary	Liver, spleen, T2* (dark)
BMS 180549	Lymph nodes	Superparamagnetic particles, T1 (bright) and T2 (dark)
DyDTPA-BMA	"Perfusion"	Susceptibility agent, dynamic/functional studies, brain and heart, no T1 effect and T2* (dark)

Table 5.5. New Contrast Agents: In the Laboratory

Agent	Application	Comments
WIN 39996	Gastro intestinal	Superparamagnetic particles, T2 (dark)
Mn(II)-HA	Hepatobiliary	Hydroxylapatite particles, T1 (bright)
Memsomes	Hepatobiliary	MnEDTA-DPP liposomes, T1 (bright)
DyDOTA-polylysine	Blood pool	Macromolecular contrast agent, T2* (dark)
GdDTPA-polylysine	Blood pool	Macromolecular contrast agent, T1 (bright)
Gd-based polymers	Blood pool	Macromolecular contrast agent, T1 (bright)
AMI-HS	Receptor specific	Liver, T1 (bright) and T2 (dark)
GdDTPA-dopamine	Receptor specific	Heart
Gd-TPPS$_4$	Tumor selective	Metalloporphyrins
^{17}O	Non-^{1}H nucleus	Direct observation using ^{17}O MR scanning or indirect observation using ^{1}H MR imaging as T2 (dark)
^{19}F	Non-^{1}H nucleus	Direct observation using ^{19}F MR scanning or indirect observation using ^{1}H MR imaging as T1 and T2 (dark)

hepatobiliary agents, susceptibility agents for dynamic/functional MRI, blood pool agents, new extracellular fluid agents, and lymphographic agents (Table 5.4). Even though these agents are being administered to patients in the setting of controlled clinical trials, none is expected to be available for routine clinical use until at least 1998.

In addition to agents that have progressed to clinical trials, numerous other agents are currently being tested for efficacy in animal models of human disease (Table 5.5). Since these agents have yet to demonstrate safety and efficacy in patients, they are unlikely to be approved for routine clinical use for at least 5 years.

Additional Reading

Brasch RC. MRI contrast enhancement in the central nervous system. New York: Raven Press 1993.

Brown ED, Semelka RC. Contrast enhanced magnetic resonance imaging of the abdomen. *Magn Resonance Q*, 10:2, 97–124 (1994).

Stark DD, Bradley WG. Magnetic resonance imaging, 2nd ed. Chicago: Mosby-Year Book, 1992, Chapter 14.

6

Clinical Applications

Since its introduction 10 or more years ago, MRI has evolved from a promising new modality to an indispensable diagnostic tool. Advances in radio frequency electronics, gradient hardware, computers, and pulse sequence techniques have made it possible to obtain images in shorter and shorter times, allowing improved image quality. Progress in clinical MRI applications has spurred the development of subspecialties within MRI. This chapter presents an overview of the techniques used in routine clinical MRI of various organs, along with selected examples.

It is ultimately the goal of any diagnostic modality to identify and differentiate abnormal tissue and processes from those that are considered normal. In this regard, the ability of MRI to provide three-dimensional anatomical information, paired with its exquisite sensitivity to the physicochemical state of tissue, is its main strength. Each type of tissue is characterized by intrinsic relaxation properties and thus a characteristic appearance on specific MR images. In practice, the characterization of a suspicious lesion or abnormality is arrived at by using a combination of pulse sequence protocols, each weighted to enhance one or more spin properties of the lesion, to observe the behavior of image contrast. The most common parameters are T1 and T2, as elaborated in Chapter 4. The introduction of intravenous paramagnetic contrast agents has added another dimension for probing the vascular properties of a given lesion.

Scan Protocols

The pulse sequence protocols used for any given application have evolved by careful consideration of spatial resolution, necessary coverage, scan time, and contrast behavior. The main parameters that compose a pulse sequence protocol are given in Table 6.1.

Table 6.1. A Typical Pulse Sequence Printout, showing the Primary MRI Parameters

pulse-sequence
  name: spin-echo###
protocol name: pelvis_####

Recycle time (TR)	Slice, phase orientation	Physiological triggering (y/n)
Echo times (TE)	Matrix size	Pre saturation (spatial, spectral)
Inversion delay (TI)	Field of view (FOV)	Half-Fourier, oversampling options
Number, position of slices	Signal averages	Filter options
Slice thickness	Bandwidth	Asymmetric FOV options
Interslice gap	Number of echoes in echo train	Post processing options

The parameters TR and TE are chosen to achieve the desired T1 and T2 image contrast. T1 weighting requires short TR and TE (500–700/15–25 ms). T2 weighting requires long TR and TE values (2000–3000/60–100 ms). T2-weighted sequences are generally constructed to generate two echoes, one with an echo time of less than 30 ms and the other a late echo at 60 ms or more. The first echo yields an image weighted by the spin density (concentration of water protons) rather than by T1 and T2 effects. The inversion delay time T1 is applicable only for inversion recovery sequence, when it is desirable to suppress a given tissue signal. An inversion time of 130–150 ms will suppress signal from fat, for example; 300–350 ms will suppress signal from silicone implants. A set of parameters allows prescription of slices and saturation regions of desired orientation, thickness, and separation, with options to set the directions for frequency and phase encoding. The other parameters, including FOV and matrix size, affect the spatial resolution of the image.

The choice of imaging planes is usually based on the familiarity of the radiologists with visualization of the anatomical structures. The readout direction is generally chosen along the long axis of the image, to prevent wraparound artifacts. Also, this choice entails fewer phase encode steps, resulting in shorter imaging time. For example, to acquire coronal images of the brain, the superior-to-inferior axis is chosen for readout and the mediolateral axis is chosen for phase-encoding coding.

With most MRI instruments, the pulse sequence protocols associated with individual organs are generally saved as computer files for easy retrieval. The positioning of the slices is generally the only step needed for image acquisition. As a rule, the prescription of slices is performed by graphically placing cursors on **scout images** that are rapidly recorded gradient-echo images, along one or more orientations about the isocenter of the magnet. Thus, proper positioning of the patient within the magnet is a critical step.

Brain

The brain is one of the most commonly imaged regions of the body, since MRI can provide excellent tissue contrast deep within the cranium. When a dedicated head coil is available, high resolution images (submillimeter resolution) can be routinely generated. A T1-weighted sagittal and a T2-weighted axial examination are integral parts of all brain scans. Additional scans are generally performed for other indications. In imaging the brain, T1-weighted images demonstrate excellent anatomic detail and are useful for the detection of fatty components and hemorrhage. The use of T1 contrast agent is indicated when disruption of the blood/brain barrier is expected (e.g., in cases of tumors, pituitary adenomas, multiple sclerosis plaques). To suppress the signal from blood vessels, gradient motion compensation is generally avoided for these scans. In addition, a thick inferior presaturation slice is turned on to suppress signal from flow-related artifacts caused by pulsating blood flow.

T2-weighted images are generally used for the visualization of pathology. T2-weighted sequences yield two or more echoes and as a rule are performed axially with flow compensation turned on. The first echo (20–30 ms) generates a proton density image with some T1 weighting mixed in. The T1-based suppression of CSF signal in these images relative to pure proton density images enhances the contrast of periventricular lesions. This is particularly important when one is using T2 imaging based on the RARE (i.e., FSE or turbo-SE) pulse sequences.

The use of fast-spin-echo approaches for T2 contrast instead of conventional spin-echo methods is becoming increasingly common. FSE sequence offer a considerable saving in time by acquiring multiple lines of data from each RF excitation. Thus, if a train of eight echoes is used to collect eight lines of data, the scan time is reduced by a factor of 8. However, FSE sequences produce altered T2 contrast as a result of echoes acquired over a range of

---

Coils for Spine Imaging   Individual surface coils are generally used for imaging the cervical, thoracic, and lumbar spinal regions, with the patient supine on the coil. More recently coil arrays have been developed, that allow entire-spine imaging without the need for switching coils.

Table 6.2. Imaging Techniques Associated with Common Brain Indications

Indications	Comments and additional sequences
Congenital anomaly and development delays	Thinner slices (4 mm) for infants and 3D imaging for multiplanar reconstruction; longer TR values to allow for increased T1 in infants
Demyelinating disease	Postcontrast scan
Stroke and hemorrhage	MRA, T2* sequence for hematoma
Tumor	Postcontrast scan
Vascular disease (AVM and aneurysms)	MRA sequences, non-flow-compensated SE sequences
Seizures: temporal lobe epilepsy	Thin-slice coronal T2 to detect hippocampal sclerosis (3 mm)
Optic neuropathy	Fat-saturated postcontrast scan
Pituitary dysfunction	Thin slice images (3 mm)

TE values. Also, fat signal appears bright in the long echo image, unlike a conventional T2-weighted image. Table 6.2 lists some of the common indications and associated comments.

In addition to the standard T1- and T2-weighted pulse sequences, scans of other types are generally used. Coronal images are required for imaging the internal auditory canal (IAC), as well as lesions of the sella and temporal lobe. Gradient-echo scans demonstrating T2* contrast are used to detect changes in magnetic susceptibility from hemorrhage. Fat suppression sequences such as STIR or chemical shift selective suppression sequences are used to lower the fat signal in imaging the orbit, thereby improving lesion contrast in T1-weighted images. Also, 3D fast-gradient-echo sequences allow the acquisition of volume data sets, which can be used in the reconstruction of images in any arbitrary plane for preoperative localization of lesions. Figure 6.1 shows T1- and T2-weighted images obtained from a patient with diffused metastatic lesions.

Spine: Cervical, Thoracic, and Lumbar

In recent years MRI has become the imaging modality of choice for studying the spine and associated structures. The other options for diagnosing pathology include computerized tomography and intrathecal injection of contrast agents. However the ability of MR to generate images of the full spine at arbitrary orientations and to provide excellent tissue contrast has made it all but indispensable for spine imaging. MRI has been found to be particularly suited for studying myelopathy and

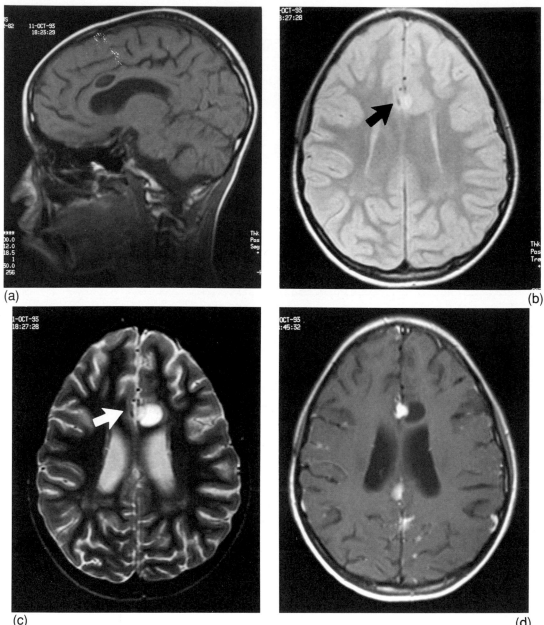

(a)

(b)

(c)

(d)

Figure 6.1. (a) Sagittal T1-weighted image showing cystic lesions superior to the ventricles in the body of the corpus callosum (arrow). (b,c) T2-weighted axial image and a proton density image showing bright lesions anterior to the ventricles in both the first and second echoes with a hint of mass to the right side of the cystic lesion (arrow). T2-weighted images also demonstrate some atrophy of the brain, evidenced by the rather enlarged ventricles. (d) Postcontrast T1-weighted images reveal enhancing lesions of leptomeningitis as well as the mass abutting the cystic lesion.

reticulopathy. In this section we examine some of the techniques used for spine imaging.

Just as for the brain, T1-weighted images provide excellent visualization of anatomical structures. CSF appears dark against the brighter signal of the cord, although gray–white matter is not resolved because of spatial resolution limits. Bony anatomy is seen clearly by the bright appearance of marrow and fat against the dark cortical bone. T1-weighted images are generally obtained in the sagittal and axial orientations, with the following scan parameters: TR = 600, TE = 15–20, FOV = 250–300 mm^2, matrix size = 256 × 256, slice = 3 mm, NEX = 3–4. Fewer phase-encode lines are needed if the FOV is rectangular. Respiratory motion artifacts are suppressed by the use of one or more presaturation RF pulses, applied anteriorly as coronal slices. As with the brain, the use of a contrast agent is indicated when disruption of the blood/brain barrier is suspected.

In addition, T2-weighted images are generally obtained in the sagittal plane. They allow visualization of lesions within the cord parenchyma, which are generally not well defined in T1 images. A bright signal is observed from CSF, since its T2 value is long with respect to the cord. The CSF pulsation can cause smearing artifacts and is best suppressed by synchronizing the data acquisition (ECG triggering) relative to the ECG signal. Lesions produced by demyelination, such as gliosis and edema, are best demonstrated in T2-weighted images. Scan parameters used typical are as follows: TR = 2000–2500 ms, TE = 20–80 ms, FOV = 250 × 250 mm^2, matrix = 256 × 256, NEX = 1–2, slice = 3–4 mm. Fast-spin-echo sequences are being increasingly used for T2-weighted scans, a modification that can considerably shorten scan time. However, diminished contrast has been noted for lesions from hemorrhage. As experience with this family of pulse sequences grows, FSE T2 scans will eventually replace the conventional scans.

Gradient-echo scans, with motion compensation, are performed in either in the axial or the sagittal plane. In axial scans, the lateral involvement of suspected pathology can be further assessed. Flip angles are small, and thus the contrast behavior observed in these scans generally resembles that of a proton density image. The thin slices offered by this method are useful for looking at intravertebral disk disease and the neural foramina. The following parameters are associated with this sequence: TR = 560 ms, TE = 10–15 ms, flip = 10–15°, FOV = 280 mm (rectangular FOV), NEX = 1, slice = 2–3 mm, and matrix = 256 × 256. With the advent of postprocessing methods such as multiplanar reconstruction (MPR), it is possible to acquire a 3D data set in the sagittal plane, with subsequent reconstruction of

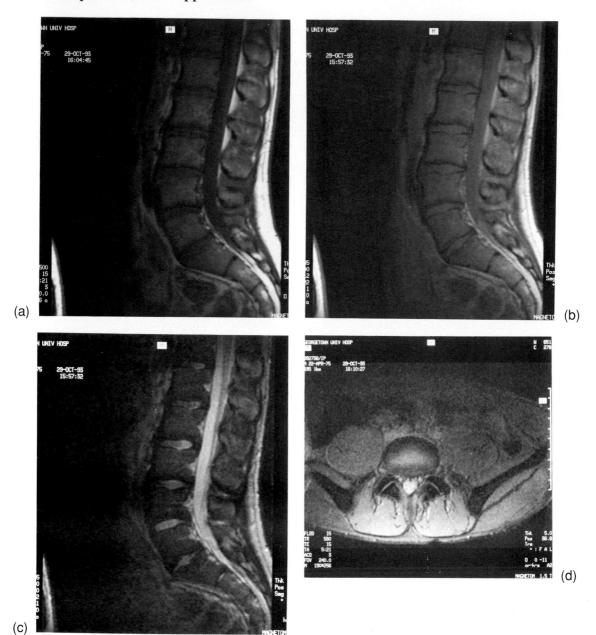

Figure 6.2. (a) T1-weighted image of the lumbar region; the CSF signal appears hypointense relative to the cord. (b) PD image of the same region; CSF is isointense relative to the cord. Although CSF has higher proton density, it does not appear brighter than cord, owing to Greater T1 weighting. (c) T2-weighted image displays brighter CSF and disk signal. (d) Axial GRE image depicting nerve roots (arrow).

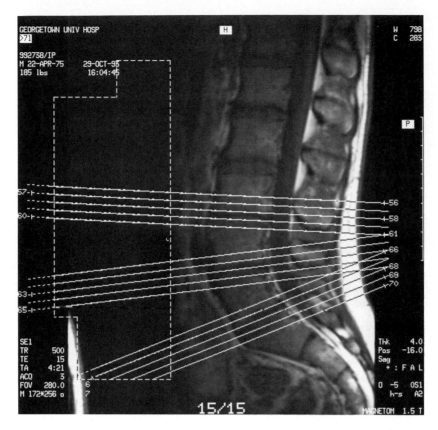

Figure 6.3. Slice prescription for transverse imaging of the lumbar spine region.

thin axial slices. Examples of spine images demonstrating pathology are shown in Figure 6.2.

In lumbar imaging, axial slices normal to the axis of spine are obtained by prescribing slices normal to the curvature of the spine. An example of such a slice prescription is shown in Figure 6.3. Some common conditions, along with special concerns relating to scan protocols, are indicated in Table 6.3.

Flow-sensitive sequences are being used increasingly to demonstrate and quantify CSF and the cord motion. This analysis is

Table 6.3. Imaging Techniques Associated with Common Spine Indications

Indication	Notes
Tumors	Pre- and postcontrast, T2
Multiple sclerosis	Pre- and postcontrast, T2
Disk herniation	Axial GRE
Spinal stenosis	T2, axial GRE
Metastasis	Full spine scan, contrast agent, matrix = 512 × 512, fat-sat

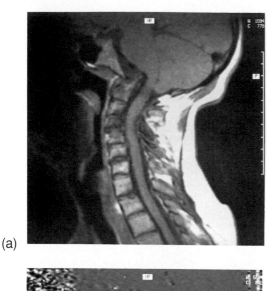

(a)

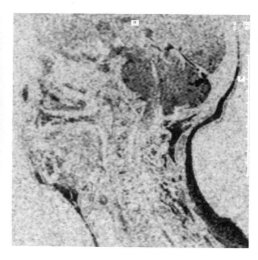

(b)

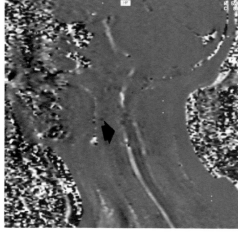

(c)

Figure 6.4. Sagittal views across a spinal cord stenosis: (a) a triggered SE magnitude image showing cord anatomy; (b) SSFP flow-sensitive sequence showing absence of flow void; (c) A phase contrast image showing absence of flow-induced phase shift at the level of the arrow.

generally performed with phase reconstruction of the raw data. Figure 6.4a is an example of a case of CSF flow constriction using an SSFP sequence; in Figure 6.4b, a phase reconstruction of a spin-echo image to used to demonstrate cord constriction.

Body Imaging: Liver, Kidney, Spleen, and Pancreas

Body imaging has been the fastest growing segment of MRI during the last 5 years. Recent advances in imaging techniques and fast imaging have made MRI a serious contender with CT and ultrasound in this area. Imaging of liver, kidney, spleen, and pancreas presents unique technical challenges. The large dimensions needed for body imaging call for larger matrix sizes to maintain a spatial resolution under 1 mm. To preserve good image quality within the FOV, adequate gradient linearity and B_0 homogeneity are needed. Problems are subject to arise in several

Table 6.4. Relaxation Times of Abdominal Tissues

Organ or tissue	Relaxation times (ms)	
	T1 (1.5T)	T2
Liver	490	43
Spleen	780	62
Muscle	870	47
Kidney	650	58
Fat	260	84

areas. The respiratory motion of the chest wall and abdomen can cause significant smearing artifacts across the image. The pulsating flow of blood in the blood vessels can cause significant artifacts across the image field. The presence of fatty structures can cause chemical shift related artifacts. And, finally, the use of the body coil for signal reception can limit the SNR of high resolution images. Most of these problems, have been successfully surmounted by the combined use of new imaging techniques and improved instrumentation.

The most commonly used pulse sequences are the T1- and T2-weighted spin-echo sequences in the transverse planes, in addition to gadolinium-enhanced, rapid gradient-echo sequences. Table 6.4 lists the T1 and T2 estimates of five major tissues. Of these, the liver is the most commonly imaged. In T1-weighted images, normal liver is bright compared to spleen, and the contrast is reversed for T2-weighted images. FSE-based, T2-weighted images have become increasingly common for body imaging because of greater savings in time and much improved image quality, despite agreement that the image contrast is altered in comparison to that of conventional spin-echo contrast. Breath-held FSE imaging also enables clear visualization of the gall bladder and the bile and pancreatic ducts. Table 6.5 gives the contrast characteristics of common liver lesions. Considerable overlap is present in the contrast behavior indicated. Therefore,

Table 6.5. The Signal Behavior of Liver Pathologies in Pre- and Postcontrast Images

	Appearance on T1	Appearance on T2	Gd uptake
Cysts	Dark	Bright	No
Hemangiomas	Dark	Bright	Variable
Hepatic adenomas	Iso-dark	Iso-bright	Fast–medium
Metastases	Variable	Variable	Heterogeneous
Cirrhosis	Variable	Variable	Slow, irregular
Fatty infiltration	Isointense	Isointense	No

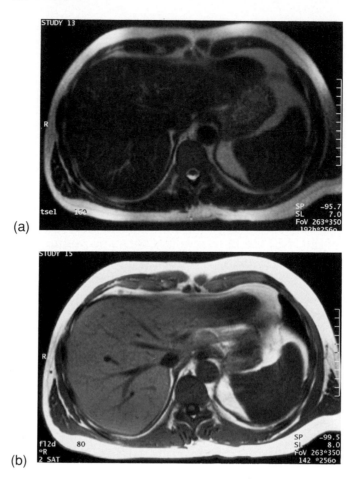

(a)

(b)

Figure 6.5. Transverse liver images recorded in one breath-hold period. (a) T1-weighted rapid gradient-echo image showing bright liver against the darker spleen. (b) T2-weighted image acquired using a half-Fourier single-shot technique.

recognizing the morphological differences becomes important in the differential diagnosis of these diseases. Figure 6.5 shows examples of a transverse section across the liver.

In evaluating the kidneys, T1-weighted SE and contrast-enhanced dynamic scans are the most widely used techniques. The T1 images show little corticomedullary differentiation, and the pancreas displays the same intensity as the kidneys. Renal images are generally acquired along the short (transverse) and long (coronal) axes of the kidneys for better delineation of anatomy. The signal behavior of lesions upon injection of contrast agent allows the characterization of these abnormalities. The characteristic signal changes within the cortex also allow functional imaging of the kidney to evaluate conditions such as renal obstruction. A breath-hold, gradient-echo scan is performed before injection of, a bolus of contrast agent, and a series of scans

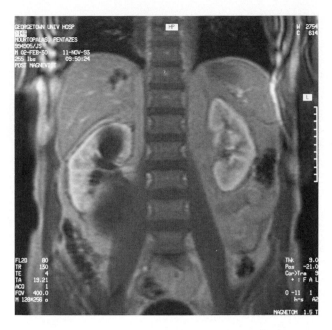

Figure 6.6. Renal cysts appear as hypointense lesions in the T1-weighted coronal sections of the kidneys.

after. The parameters used are TR = 130 ms, TE = 4 ms, 11 slices, matrix = 256 × 128, flip angle = 80° and rectangular FOV = 400 × 300 mm². Figure 6.6 shows a series of images recorded during a typical dynamic MR study of a patient with renal cysts. Note the early enhancement of the kidneys relative to liver and spleen.

During this period there is excellent corticomedullary differentiation, which gradually diminishes. Concurrently, an increase in the signal from spleen is followed by a rise in the signal from liver. The cystic regions remain unenhanced. In contrast to cysts, lesions originating from renal cell carcinoma display rapid enhancements. Enhancing lesions are frequently followed up with fat-saturated gradient-echo scans to better visualize the margins of the lesions.

As in the kidney, postcontrast gradient-echo scans are vital for the detection of lesions in the spleen as well as in the pancreas. In most instances, these dynamic scans are performed after a set of routine T1- and T2-weighted scans. The pancreas is best visualized as a bright structure using fat-suppressed spin-echo sequences. Pancreatic tumors and pancreatitis lesions generally appear as hypointense lesions (Figure 6.7).

Great Vessels and Cardiac Imaging

Imaging of the heart and the great vessels presents unique challenges to MRI and at the same time could benefit most from the

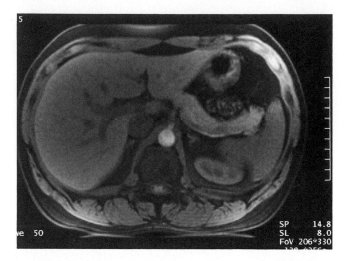

Figure 6.7. Normal pancreas anatomy shown using a water excitation, T1-weighted gradient-echo scan.

noninvasive, multiplanar capabilities of MRI. Accurate imaging of the heart has to overcome artifacts from the pulsatile motion of the organ and the slower motion due to respiration. On the other hand, the ability to noninvasively image the anatomy in any arbitrary plane, combined with the technical advances in rapid imaging, has made MRI a clinically useful tool.

Echocardiography, which is also a noninvasive technique, is still the method of choice for reasons of cost and portability. Ultrasound penetration constraints, however, make it difficult to examine regions deep within the body. X-ray-based cardiac angiography, long the gold standard, also presents significant risks. In addition to anatomic imaging, recent advances

---

Myocardial Spin Tagging   The motion patterns of the myocardial walls can be be studied by the MRI technique known as myocardial tagging. The acronyms associated with this technique are SPAMM (spatial modulation of magnetization) and STAG (spatial tagging). At the beginning of each cardiac cycle (R-wave trigger), the positions of the myocardial walls are tagged by means of presaturation pulses. These are essentially slice-selective routines applied orthogonal to the imaging plane. The presaturation pulses produce a grid of signal-void regions on the spin-echo or gradient echo cine image. During the course of the cycle, movement patterns of the myocardial regions manifest as distortions of the saturation grid, which allow the detection of functional deficits of the myocardium.

allow for assessment of blood flow, perfusion, and cardiac wall motion.

The motion of the cardiac and vascular structures during the cardiac cycle poses a major problem in imaging the heart and the great vessels. A conventional MRI scan would result in an image with smearing of the moving regions across the phase-encode direction. This is because the moving pixels are in different positions for each line of data. Fortunately, the cardiac motion is periodic in most instances, and there is minimal motion during the end-systole and end-diastole parts of the cardiac cycle. By synchronizing the onset of MR data acquisition to the cardiac cycle (R wave), all the phase-encode lines comprising the data matrix will see identically displaced regions. This implies that an image comprising 128 phase-encode lines of data will take at least 128 heartbeats for the completion of the scan. Such a procedure, known as an electrocardiograph-triggered scan, useful for imaging not only the heart and great vessels but also the spine, CSF, and arteries. The other approach to eliminating motion-related artifacts is the use of ultrafast imaging methods such as echo-planar imaging, and spiral-imaging.

Two types of pulse sequence have found use in cardiac MRI. These are the short-TE, multislice spin-echo and the flow-compensated, cine-mode, gradient-echo sequences. The spin-echo sequences are designed to show the anatomical features of the myocardium, the fat layers, and the lumina of the vessels while suppressing signal from flowing medium. With this sequence, fat appears bright, myocardium is medium gray, and blood appears dark. The imaging planes used in cardiac imaging are the long and short axes of the heart. The long axis of the heart is the one that coincides with the axis connecting the base and apex of the heart. This axis is achieved by double-tilting relative to the sagittal imaging plane. The short axis is made to be orthogonal to the long axis. Examples of ECG-triggered images of the myocardium along the short and long axis of the heart appear in Figure 6.8.

The imaging plane most useful for imaging the aorta is the left anterior oblique (LAO) plane. In this plane the entire segment from the ascending aorta through the arch to the descending part of the vessel is visible. This technique is useful for the evaluation of congenital defects. In most instances transverse and coronal images are also acquired to map the anatomical layout of the major vessels.

The spin-echo scans are usually performed in the multislice mode. This means that the various slices are acquired at different parts of the cardiac cycle and therefore do not reflect the true slice positions as seen on the slice prescription. Another caveat

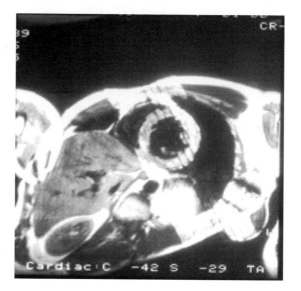

(a)

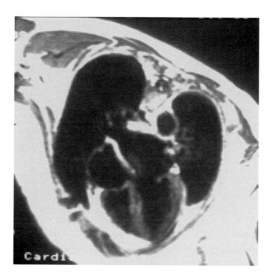

(b)

Figure 6.8. Short (a) and long axis (b) axes of the heart. (Courtesy of Dr. Curfis Green.)

Table 6.6. Commonly Used Parameters in Spin-Echo and GRE Cardiac Imaging

	TR/TE/Flip (deg)	Slice Thickness (mm)	Number of averages	Matrix	FOV (mm^2)
Spin echo, dark blood	500/30/90–180	10	3	128×256	350
GRE, bright blood	50/12/50	5–7	3	128×256	350

pertains to the TR value of an ECG-triggered scan. Since the data acquisition is triggered, the actual TR value will correspond to the mean value of the time between two consecutive R waves of the patient's ECG. To trigger the scan for every R wave, the operator enters a TR parameter that is approximately 75% of the R–R interval. If the requested value of TR happens to exceed the R–R interval in a given instance, scanning will not begin until the subsequent R wave (after the TR period) has occurred. This will prolong the scan time and may cause blurring. Choosing too low a value of TR will reduce the number of slices that can be imaged. Hence a judicious choice of TR needs to be made for maximum efficiency.

The cine-mode, gradient-echo scan is generally performed to observe the temporal changes at a given slice position. Temporal resolution may be traded for additional slices. As in most GRE sequences, the in-flow effect produces intense signal from flowing blood (refer to Chapter 7 on flow imaging). Also, the short repetition time ensures saturation of stationary structures. These are used for evaluation of blood flow patterns and functional imaging. Table 6.6 gives typical values of the scan protocol parameters for imaging the heart. The field of cardiac MRI is rapidly progressing, propelled by improvements in instrument hardware for rapid imaging. Some areas that will see greater use of MR are (a) the use of contrast agents to evaluate myocardial infarction and perfusion, (b) MR coronary angiography, (c) ultrafast cardiac imaging, and (d) velocity mapping by means of phase measurements.

Breast Imaging

The use of MRI for screening of breast cancer (BMRI) and the evaluation of breast implants has received much interest recently. Breast imaging is difficult because breast tissue is mostly fatty, and therefore conventional spin-echo imaging would necessitate additional fat suppression schemes. On early MRI systems this was not always possible, since field homogeneity was not always satisfactory. Also, the high spatial resolution needed for breast imaging cannot be obtained when the body coil is used, and this limitation has led to the development of dedicated breast coils. The most common coil configuration is a pair of coil wells built into the cushion. The patient is imaged lying prone on the coil.

These has been considerable interest recently in the use of dynamic GRE imaging, enhanced by contrast agent, in the detection of breast cancer lesions. This technique is sensitive enough to detect lesions 2–3 mm in size, even without the use of fat suppression. Rapid GRE images, covering the entire breast, are performed before and several times after a bolus of gadolinium-based contrast agent. The temporal response of the uptake of the contrast agent, as measured by the increased signal, is used for the evaluation of lesions. Despite the sensitivity of this technique, many questions remain about its specificity for screening

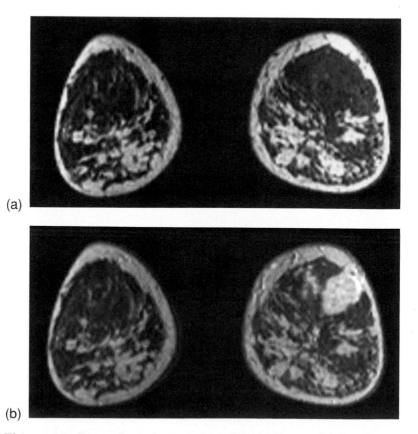

(a)

(b)

Figure 6.9. Examples of coronal rapid gradient-echo breast images precontrast (a) and postcontrast (b). Note enhancing lesion at upper left quadrant in left breast.

purposes. Figure 6.9 shows series of images from a patient suspected of having a breast mass, before and after administration of contrast agent.

The introduction of biopsy devices that can be used in conjunction with MRI is certain to be of enormous help in breast cancer detection. Despite the low specificity, BMRI has been found to be useful in the imaging of patients with mammographically dense breasts.

MRI is also the method of choice for the evaluation of the integrity of breast implants. There are two major health issues associated with the use of silicone implants: the reduced efficacy of conventional mammography in women with implants (due primarily to the high radiopacity of the silicone gel contained in the implant) and the long-term effects attributed to such implants. There is considerable risk that the rubber envelope will be ruptured by the body's digestive enzymes. In addition, silicone has been found to seep to regions outside the rubber envelope.

MRI of breast implants is complicated by the numerous types of implant that have been used for augmentation. Most of these devices have one or more compartments containing silicone and saline. The imaging problem reduces to one of obtaining sufficient contrast between silicone, water, and fat. Also, 3D volume data has been found to be helpful in inferring the contours of the implant. A transverse image set is first obtained to evaluate the implants for overall shape, size, and type. This is usually followed by one or more component-selective scans, such as fat- or silicone-selective scans. Inversion recovery or chemical shift selective saturation generally is used in combination with FSE based sequences. A rapid 3D gradient echo scan is also performed to get thin-slice volume data, which allows reconstruction of images along arbitrary planes for better visualization of contours. Imaging yields information on the integrity of the fibrous capsule surrounding the rubber envelope, and the extent of the silicone migration.

Figure 6.10 shows examples of images from a patient with bilateral silicone implants. An FOV of 37.5×37.5 cm, a slice thickness of 5 mm, and a 256×512 data matrix are generally used for transverse and coronal images. Figure 6.10a is a T1-weighted image showing hyperintense signal from silicone and fibrous capsule and medium-intense signal from glandular tissue; the most intense signal is from fat. A T2-weighted FSE scan with inversion pulse shows brightest signal from silicone, with adequate fat suppression occurring at an inversion delay time of 100 ms (Figure 6.10b). The images from the steady state sequence (Figure 6.10c) allow the visualization of the boundaries of the implants.

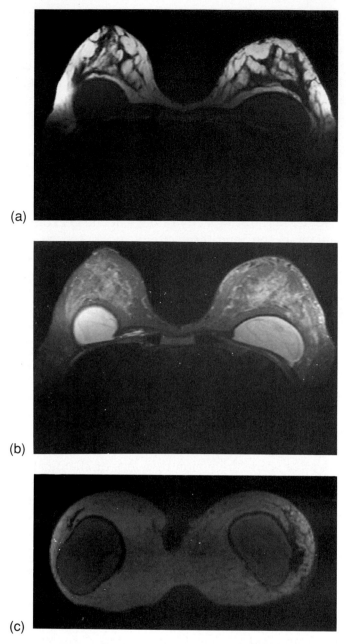

(a)

(b)

(c)

Figure 6.10. Transverse images of bilateral silicone implants. (a) T1-weighted image showing bright fatty structures. (b) Inversion recovery method. (c) Steady state gradient-echo method.

Musculoskeletal Imaging

Imaging of the knee, shoulder, wrist, elbow, and ankle are also well accomplished with MRI. Each of these regions presents its own set of technical challenges. The need for submillimeter spatial resolution, the complexity of joint anatomy, the variety of tissue types, and the location and shape of the joints have contributed to the difficulty of imaging these regions of the body. Most of the technical challenges have been successfully overcome in recent years, and MRI is now the method of choice for studying joint injuries and musculoskeletal tumors because of its versatility in garnering three-dimensional information, as well as the superior soft-tissue contrast.

The eccentric location of the shoulder and wrist joints has been the major impediment to their imaging. Improved instrument capabilities are needed to selectively image regions placed away from the center of the magnet, as in the case of a shoulder joint. Figure 6.11 shows an example of a shoulder scout image covering the entire region about the center of the magnet as well the

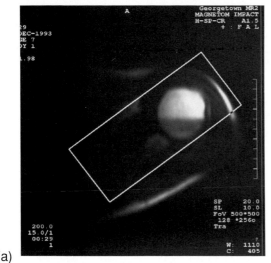

(a)

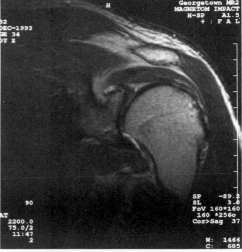

(b)

Figure 6.11. (a) Larger FOV scout image of the shoulder. (b) High resolution T1-weighted image of the shoulder. (c) T2-weighted image of the shoulder displaying bright signal from fluid collection around the joint.

(c)

zoomed-in high resolution image. Since, a 15 cm FOV typically is imaged using a matrix size of 256×256, an efficient local coil is essential for adequate SNR.

Spin-echo T1- and T2-weighted imaging is routinely performed for the visualization of joint anatomy. Injury to ligaments and tendons is easily visualized as increased signal. A common application in which MRI has proven to be extremely sensitive is the grading of meniscal tears in the knee joint. The presence of synovial fluid is readily detected using T2-weighted imaging. However, the bright fat signal present in T2-weighted FSE scans can obscure fat/fluid boundaries and has led to the use of fat presaturation for these applications. In addition, 3D gradient-echo sequences are generally included in imaging protocols to allow the visualization of anatomy in any arbitrary plane. This has been a particularity valuable asset for MR in the imaging of musculoskeletal regions, with their complex joint anatomy. Figure 6.12 shows an example of ankle images obtained from a 3D gradient-echo scan.

Pelvic Imaging

Just as in the liver, leaps in the capability of MRI hardware have contributed to the successful imaging of the pelvis. Unlike abdominal imaging, however, the visualization of pelvic anatomic structures generally requires submillimeter spatial resolution. The advent of sensitive phased-array coils has allowed routine imaging of the prostate, uterus, cervix, and associated organs whose zonal anatomy is best visualized in T2-weighted images of thin slices (<3 mm). FSE pulse sequences are generally used to maximize signal.

The customary protocols for imaging the prostate comprise (a) T1- and T2-weighted high resolution images in the transverse direction to cover the prostate gland, (b) T2-weighted high resolution sagittal images, and (c) T1-weighted transverse images, with coarse matrix, to cover the entire pelvis. The whole-pelvis scan is used for screening the lymph nodes for involvement of cancer. The prostate gland generally appears hyperintense and isointense in T2- and T1-weighted images, respectively, relative to cancerous lesions. Associated structures, such as the seminal vesicles, neurovascular bundle, rectum, and bladder can also be observed. An example of a transverse section of the prostate is depicted in Figure 6.13.

MRI is particularly suited for the diagnosis of adenomyosis, endometriomas, carcinomas, cysts, leiomyomas, and polyps. High resolution T1- and T2-weighted images in the transverse and sagittal orientations are generally performed. In addition,

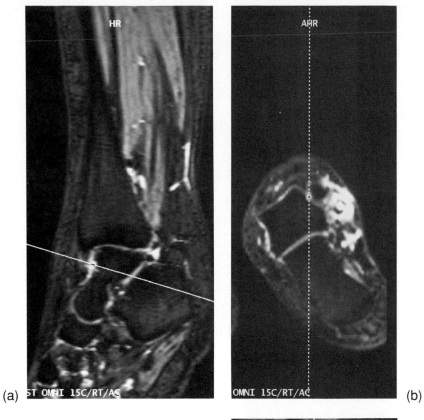

(a)

(b)

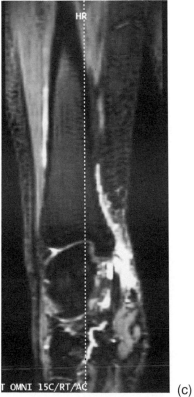

Figure 6.12. Example of a 3D GRE scan depicting the raw image (a) as well as the images reconstructed along the orthogonal planes from the 3D data set (b,c).

(c)

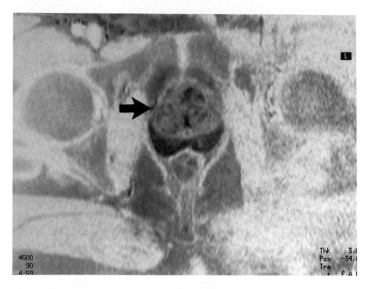

Figure 6.13. T2-weighted transverse images across the prostate gland. Note the bright signal behavior from gland (arrow), in contrast to the inner zone.

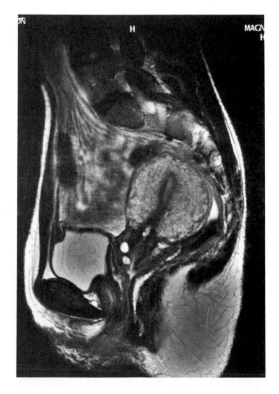

Figure 6.14. T2-weighted sagittal image depicting normal zonal anatomy of the uterus (arrow).

postcontrast scans are performed for differential diagnosis, An example of a sagittal image depicting the zonal anatomy of the uterus and cervix appears in Figure 6.14.

This chapter has presented merely a glimpse of the myriad clinical applications of MRI. With continuing improvements in imaging technology, newer applications are sure to follow. In addition, clinical outcome studies will ultimately direct the judicious use of MR toward the ever expanding number of applications.

Additional Reading

Edelman RR, Hesselink JR, eds. Clinical magnetic resonance imaging. Philadelphia: WB Saunders Company, 199.

Stark DD, Bradley WG. Magnetic resonance imaging, 2nd ed. Chicago: Mosby-Yea Book, 1992.

Wood M, Bronskill M. MR desktop data. *J Magn Resonance Imaging* 2(S):13–17 (1992).

7

Flow Effects and MR Angiography

As described in Chapter 6, the choice of imaging parameters and the spin properties of the tissue determine the intensity of the MR signal and the resulting image contrast for a stationary medium. Ultimately it is the steady state values of the longitudinal magnetization and the resulting transverse magnetization during the detection period that will provide the signal. Blood is a composed of cellular and noncellular components and is about 80% water by weight. Therefore stationary blood will produce a signal similar to other tissue with long T1 and T2. In the presence of flow, the M_x, M_y, and M_z magnetizations are further modified to produce a variety of effects (flow void, flow saturation, ghosting, etc.), depending on the imaging pulse sequence and scan parameters. Before we examine these effects, it is important to understand the nature of blood flow in vessels.

The flow of blood in any given region of the body will depend on a number of factors such as lumen size of the vessel, back pressure present in the tissue, pulsatile forces exerted by the heart, viscosity of the blood, and elasticity of the vessels. Other types of flow relevant to MR studies are those of cerebrospinal fluid, sinuses, and lymphatic fluids. The volume of liquid flowing through the vessel per unit time V is proportional to the expression given in equation 7.1:

$$(\text{radius of lumen})^4 \times (\text{pressure differential}) \times \left(\frac{1}{\text{viscosity}}\right) \quad (7.1)$$

The pressure difference is generated by the pumping motion of the heart. The velocity of the blood flow in all major vessels will pulsate in unison with the heart, with varying degrees of delay in time. The back pressure present in the organs can cause a delayed reflection of the forces. This effect produces a periodic reversal in flow direction in some vessels during part of the cardiac cycle. The flow dynamics is further complicated by the velocity dependence of viscosity of blood. As the velocity of blood decreases, the viscosity increases markedly, causing a tendency to form a thrombus.

Although the volume of blood transported, in units of volume per second, will determine the nutritional status of the organ, the velocity of blood, in units of distance over time, and the changes in velocity during the cardiac cycle will ultimately affect the observed MR signal. The volume of liquid flowing through a cross section per unit time is given by the product of the velocity and the cross-sectional area of the lumen. According to Bernoulli's principle, the flow volume rates at all points along the segment are of equal value, even if the cross-sectional areas vary from point to point, as shown in Figure 7.1. Therefore, velocities along the segment will depend on the cross-sectional areas at the various points. According to this principle, the velocity will vary inversely with the cross section of the lumen, assuming that the volume of blood being transported is unchanged. Such is the case when the lumen is constricted locally, as in an atherosclerotic stenosis.

Listed in Table 7.1 are the velocity ranges in some normal vessels; these are mean values, and the instantaneous velocities are a function of the phase of the cardiac cycle as well as the exact position within the lumen. The velocities are close to zero near the vessel wall and are at maximum in the center of the lumen. The flow velocities in veins and lymphatic vessels, however, are less pulsatile. The MRI signal is exquisitely sensitive to flow, and this property can be exploited to noninvasively measure flow. Flow velocities as low as a few millimeters to as high as a few meters per second can be estimated routinely.

Bernoulli's principle: $(\text{Flow rate})_{in} = (\text{Flow rate})_{out}$
Flow rate = volume/time
$\qquad$ = length x Area of Lumen / time
$\qquad$ = Vâ 1/4 $(\pi * V * d^2)$
$\qquad$ = Velocit * area
$\qquad$ = $V * (1/4) \cdot \pi \cdot d^2$

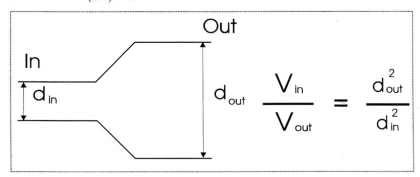

Figure 7.1. Bernoulli's flow principle, where V_{in}/V_{out} refers to the ratio of the flow velocities.

Table 7.1. Mean Velocities of Blood Flow in Some Vessel Types

Vessel type	Mean velocity (cm/s)
Internal carotid	35
Common carotid	30
Portal vein	20
Popliteal	10
Renal artery	40
Abdominal aorta	15

Flow Effects

When the direction of flow is perpendicular to the imaging plane, two distinct effects are produced. The first, a wash-in effect, will tend to alter the effective TR of the flowing spins. The second, a washout effect, will tend to decrease the signal from the flowing spins within the slice. These two effects will be examined for several special instances. Although they are strongest when the flow direction is normal to the imaging plane, they can occur whenever flow is present along any direction.

In conventional single-slice imaging, the flowing spins are relatively unsaturated compared to the stagnant spins because of the inflow effect during every TR period (Figure 7.2). Thus, the effective TR of the flowing spins in the slice being imaged will be longer because these spins, unlike the stationary spins, are not exposed to the same cycle of RF pulses. In other words, the signal enhancement will be proportional to the fraction of fresh spins populating the slice during every TR period. Maximum signal enhancement is attained when all the spins within the slice are replaced by unsaturated flowing spins during every TR period. This will occur if the distance traversed by the spins during the TR period (given by vTR) is equal to the slice thickness; for example, for a velocity of 20 cm/s and a slice thickness of 5 mm, a maximum in flow enhancement will occur with a TR of 25 ms. In principle, velocity measurements may be made by determining the TR for maximum enhancement and a known value of the slice thickness. However, the pulsatile nature of blood flow precludes the use of this technique. In conventional multislice imaging, inflow signal enhancement will affect only the first slice that contains unsaturated spins for every phase-encoded line of data. The other slices will display variable flow signal.

Under some circumstances, flow can produce a signal loss due to washout during the time course of the echo time. The spins in any given slice contribute to echo formation only if they have experienced all the RF excitation pulses and gradient pulses that form the pulse sequence. The stationary spins in the slice will experience the RF and gradient pulses and will therefore form the echo. Because of translation of the spins through the slice being imaged, however, flowing spins may not experience the same RF pulses and magnetic field pulses. This discrepancy will cause an incomplete formation of the echo and a corresponding decrease in the pixel intensity of the flowing spins.

The loss of signal due to washout is proportional to the velocity of flow and the length of the echo time. This signal loss is minimal in gradient-echo sequences because echo times are relatively short. But spin-echo sequences can suffer from significant signal losses if spins within a slice move out of the slice before the 180° refocusing pulse is turned on, as shown in Figure 7.3.

In this example the flow velocity in the top row is twice that of ($\frac{Sl}{TE}$). The part of the flowing medium that was affected by the 90° RF pulse has passed completely out of the slice before the 180° pulse is turned on. Thus no echo signal is possible from the flowing spins. When the velocity is decreased by half, the echo is formed from half the sample within the slice, as shown in the middle row of Figure 7.3. Full signal is generated in the absence of flow, as seen in the bottom row. For example, a total signal void in a 5mm thick image, obtained with a TE of 80ms, indicates a mean flow velocity of approximately 13cm/s.

In addition to the effects discussed above, flow alters the phase of the MR signal. The concept of phase of the spin vector was introduced in Chapter 3 in the description of phase and frequency encoding. The notion of phase and related concepts such as phase shifts, phase dispersion, and phase coherence will be examined again in the context of flow effects.

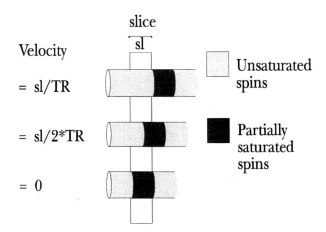

Figure 7.2. Velocity dependence of signal due to slice inflow effects.

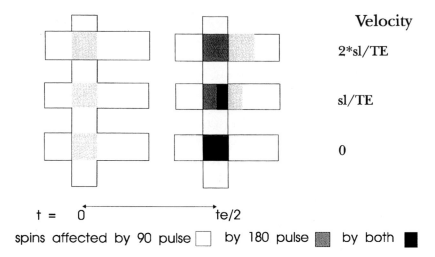

Figure 7.3. Signal loss due to slice outflow in a spin-echo pulse sequence.

The spin-phase effect is best understood by examining the dynamics of the spin vectors constituting a pixel (or voxel). Each pixel is composed of a rather a large number of spin vectors (10^{20}), and it is the vectorial sum of these vectors that is ultimately responsible for the signal intensity of each pixel in the image. In addition, each pixel is characterized by a distinct combination of Larmor frequency and phase frequency in the image derived from the resultant of all its constituent spin vectors.

During a typical MRI scan, the spin vectors first experience an RF excitation followed by evolution during the phase and frequency encode periods. Under ideal conditions, all the spin vectors comprising the pixel will evolve together to form the echo signal. This is demonstrated in Figure 7.4 for the case of three spin vectors comprising a pixel. The maximum signal is produced in this example by the vectorial addition of the parallel vectors.

However, under normal circumstances this is not the case because the spin vectors in a voxel possess a distribution of precessional frequencies, as shown in Figure 7.4, resulting in progressive dispersion of the spin vectors during echo formation. Vectorial addition of these vectors will generate a smaller signal than is found in the ideal situation described before. This phenomenon is referred to as phase dispersion.

The process of T2 relaxation is a natural mechanism that always contributes to some degree of phase dispersion, leading to image contrast. As we shall see later in this chapter, other causes such as motion, flow, and T2* can also result in loss of pixel intensity. In summary, phase dispersion of a pixel's isochromats, during echo formation, causes signal loss.

Spurious phase shifts can be caused by movement of spins along (or against) the direction of an applied field gradient. This is the basis for the rest of the flow-related effects to be described in this chapter. In Chapter 3 we learned that the phase shift induced in stationary spins is given by the product of the strength of the gradient, the time period, and the position of the spins under consideration. The position-dependent phase shift thus provides the basis for phase encoding. If the spin vectors are moving during the gradient pulse, the phase shifts will no longer be a just a linear function of time; they will depend, as well, on the velocity. If the isochromats move in the direction of higher magnetic field, the phase shifts will progressively increase relative to stationary spins, and vice versa.

To calculate the cumulative phase shift for moving spins, a general expression can be derived. The phase change during any infinitesimally small time period dt can be written as

$$d\phi = \gamma G_z z \, dt \qquad (7.2)$$

where G_z is the magnitude of the z- gradient pulse and z is the instantaneous position along the z axis. The variable z, which is a function of time, can be written as

$$z = z_0 + vt + at^3 \qquad (7.3)$$

where z_0 is the z value at the beginning of the gradient pulse, v the velocity, and a the acceleration of moving spins. After substituting the expression for z in equation 7.2, we can obtain the cumulative phase shift by integrating the expression over the time period of the gradient pulse.

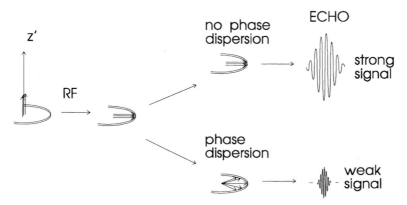

Figure 7.4. Phase dispersion within a voxel leads to signal loss.

$$\int d\phi = \int \gamma G_z \left(z_0 + vt + at^3\right)dt \qquad (7.4)$$

therefore,

$$\phi = \gamma G_z \left(z_0 t + \frac{vt^2}{2} + \frac{at^3}{3}\right)$$

Equation 7.4 shows that in the presence of flow, the phase evolution depends nonlinearly on time and on the direction of flow. This principle is illustrated in Figure 7.5, which shows the phase evolution during a gradient pulse for five different spin vectors, of which three are stationary at 1, 0, and −1 cm away from the isocenter along the z axis. The spins located at isocenter experience no phase shift. The ones located at 1 and −1 experience linear phase shift with time (only the first term in the equation contributes). The other two cases correspond to phase evolution for moving spins with velocities +v, −v. Note the nonlinear increase in phase.

The flow-induced phase shift discussed in the preceding section has several important implications:

- Any degree of pulsatility (along any of the three gradient directions) will cause spurious changes in phase from view to view. This will produce signals with new phase frequency values in the raw data, which will manifest as ghost images in the phase-encode direction.

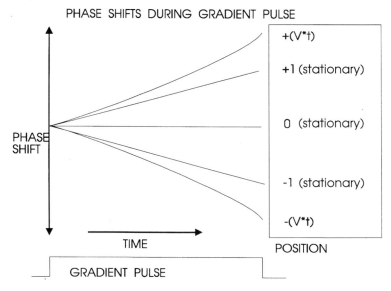

Figure 7.5. Phase shifts experienced by spin isochromats during a field gradient pulse in the presence of motion. Phase evolution is shown for five different spin vectors in the column labeled "position."

Isochromats In discussing the phase behavior of spins within a pixel, it is convenient to represent all the spins evolving together (with the same phase) with a single vector. Such a vector is a termed an isochromat. It is assumed that negligible phase dispersion occurs within the vectors comprising the isochromat. However, the isochromats themselves will undergo phase dispersion by one of the other mechanisms.

- If the isochromats constituting the pixel experience different phase shifts that are due to different velocities, additional phase dispersion occurs and, consequently, signal loss. It also follows that this mechanism of signal loss will increase with increasing pixel dimensions. For this reason, 3D scans with small pixels ($1 \times 1 \times 1\,\mathrm{mm}^3$) are preferred to 2D scans ($1 \times 1 \times 3\,\mathrm{mm}^3$) in flow imaging.
- The phase changes due to flow can be exploited to quantitatively measure flow velocities.

Flow and Motion Compensation Techniques

The preceding section revealed that moving spins experience undesirable phase shifts, which can produce signal-robbing ghost artifacts along the phase-encode direction. These spurious phase shifts can be minimized by techniques described below. The first step in addressing motion artifacts is to understand the sources of motion and the relative time scales.

Physical movement of the patient during the scanning period is perhaps the most common source of ghost artifacts. This motion is random and cannot be fully compensated for. For scans lasting less than 10 minutes, this source of motion usually does not degrade image quality significantly. Except in the most cooperative patients, however, patient motion is likely to cause artifacts if scan times exceed 10–15 minutes.

Movement of the chest wall due to respiration is another common source of artifact. The scan time of one or more minutes is rather long compared to the respiratory time scale, which is of the order of seconds. The intense fat signal from the anterior chest wall will experience movement induced phase shifts, leading to ghosts along the phase-encode direction. In the absence of some form of motion suppression, the rather intense ghost signals will obscure the region of interest. A straightforward method of rectifying this is to synchronize acquisition of data with respiratory motion. Yet another method that can be used to minimize ghost artifacts is based on the premise that, upon signal averaging, the ghosts generated from random motion will

Cardiac triggering and respiratory gating Unacceptable motion artifacts are encountered in imaging the heart and great vessels. The motion problem from the heart is circumvented by synchronizing the acquisition of data (each phase-encode line) with the ECG signal. This procedure, referred to as cardiac triggering, can be used to obtain images through the various stages of the cardiac cycle. Respiratory gating minimizes motion artifacts in body imaging applications. In this method, the respiration is monitored using a pressure transducer, while the acquisition is in progress. All data that fall outside a predefined respiration window are rejected. Although cardiac triggering is routinely used for heart imaging, scan time constraints have prevented widespread use of respiratory gating.

not add coherently like the nonghost signal and will therefore improve the image quality. However, the signal averaging approach also will lead to increased scan times. Breath-hold imaging is the most commonly used technique to image regions of the body affected by respiration such as liver and kidney, In this approach an entire set of 20 images are acquired within a breath-hold period (20–30 seconds).

The problem of motion is most acute in imaging the heart and surrounding vessels. Significant movement of the myocardium occurs in tens of milliseconds. Such rapid motion of the beating heart during image acquisition will render the image unusable if flow compensation is not augmented by some form of synchronization scheme.

Flow compensation techniques are useful in minimizing the artifacts generated by pulsatile blood flow during the imaging of stationary tissue as well as in preserving flow signal when blood vessels are being imaged. The two most common methods of increasing flow signal are called even-echo rephasing and gradient motion refocusing (GMR).

Even-echo rephasing, a simple method of correcting for flow-related phase dispersion, is achieved by the use of refocusing RF pulses, such as in a symmetric double-echo pulse sequence. Although this technique is rarely used in actual practice, it is nonetheless a useful exercise in understanding flow effects. Consider the phase evolution of a isochromat, flowing along the direction of the read gradient, as shown in Figure 7.6. The pulse sequence consists of a spin echo formed by a 90–180–180 RF pulse train (first row). During the echo periods, gradient pulses are turned on along the frequency-encode direction, as shown in the second row. In the absence of flow, the first echo signal will be formed between the 180° pulses and the second one at half-echo period after the second 180° pulse, as shown in the third row. The phase evolution is shown by the position of the vectors in the *xy* plane of the rotating coordinate system for both the stationary and moving spins. The phase evolution can also be visualized from a plot of phase shift versus time for the two isochromats.

For the stationary spins, the phase shift caused by the first gradient pulse is precisely equal but opposite in sign to the shift caused during the first half of the second gradient pulse. The result is a refocusing of the stationary spins in the center of the second gradient pulse period. By the same reasoning, the stationary spins will refocus for the second time during the center of the third gradient pulse period.

For the moving spins, however, the phase shift accumulated during the first half of the echo is not compensated by the second half of the echo. This is because the moving spins are experiencing a progressively increasing Larmor frequency relative to the stationary spins. The 180° pulses have the effect of flipping the sign of the phase shift. The net result is that the moving spins have experienced a phase gain at the end of the first echo period. Just as in the first TE period, the moving spins experience unequal phase shifts during the second TE period. However, the

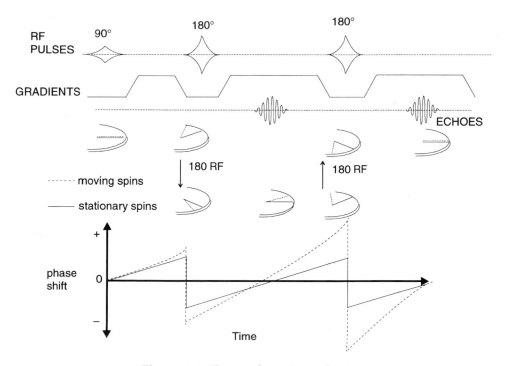

Figure 7.6. Even echo spin rephasing.

phase gain from the first echo will equal the phase loss from the second echo period. This results in complete refocusing of the moving spins during the second echo, assuming that the velocity is constant during the pulse train. By the same line of reasoning, it can be predicted that the echo formed after an odd number of 180° pulses will show decreased flow signal and that after an even number of 180° pulses, flow signal enhancement.

Other factors will alter the degree of this enhancement. The velocity of the moving spins during the two echo periods must remain constant, the intravoxel phase dispersion must be small relative to the phase shift effects, the echo times and gradient waveforms must be symmetrically placed as in the example above, and only spins moving along the direction of the gradients will display this effect. Although hard to use for reducing flow artifacts, this effect is helpful is for differentiating thrombus from flowing spins in spin-echo images.

Although the even-echo rephasing method can be useful in some instances, it is not applicable to gradient echo pulse sequences because of the absence of a 180° refocusing pulse. The gradient motion refocusing (GMR) method can be used to compensate for the net phase shift experienced by moving spins by using appropriately tailored gradient pulses. This method is also known as gradient moment nulling.

The GMR concept can be qualitatively understood by considering the phase evolution of a moving isochromat (after a 90° flip on to the $x'y'$ frame) during the application of a bipolar gradient pulse form. A bipolar gradient pulse consists of two gradient pulses, applied sequentially along the same direction, that are opposite in sign and of equal magnitude. Figure 7.7 depicts the results of applying two such bipolar gradient pulses. On the top are phase evolution plots of the stationary and moving spin vectors during a +− bipolar pulse. At the bottom are those for the −+ bipolar gradient pair. Vector representations of the spins on the $x'y'$ plane are also shown at the beginning and end of each of the gradient pulses.

Consider first the +− pulse pair. By the end of the first pulse, the moving isochromat has gained in phase relative to the stationary ones as a result of movement in the direction of increasing field. During the second gradient pulse, the spins are moving in the direction of decreasing field relative to a stationary spin, since the polarity of the gradient has reversed. This will have the effect of reversing the phase gain. At the end of the second pulse, the stationary spin isochromats will have precisely refocused, unlike the moving isochromats, which have experienced a net phase loss. This is because the phase gain that occurs during the

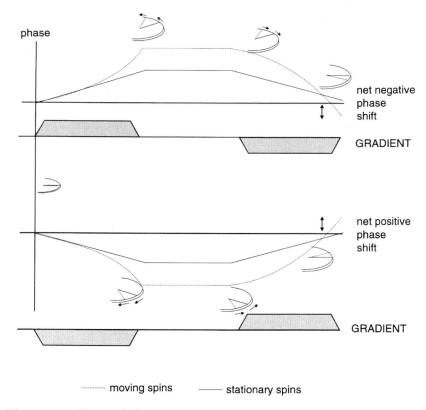

Figure 7.7. Phase shift produced in moving spins in the presence of a bipolon gradient pulse.

first pulse is less than the phase loss during the second pulse. This phase shift is a function of velocity and can be used to measure velocities, as will be explained later in this chapter. If the sign of the gradient pulses were reversed in the preceding example, the moving spins would instead have gained in phase at the end of (bipolar pulse, −+) sequence.

This line of reasoning can be extended to understand the effect of applying two bipolar pulses, +− and −+, in tandem. The phase loss produced by the first bipolar pair will compensate for the phase gain due to the second bipolar pair, leading to refocusing of moving spins for all velocities. The stationary spins will also refocus because no phase shift was generated during either bipolar pair. This mechanism is described schematically in Figure 7.8.

The concept can be extended to rephase accelerating spins too, or to selectively rephase stationary, velocity, or acceleration components. GMR is widely used in routine imaging and angiography techniques. Blood flow is always accompanied by pulsation, causing periodic changes in the velocity of the blood. Phase shifts due to pulsatile blood flow cannot be fully compen-

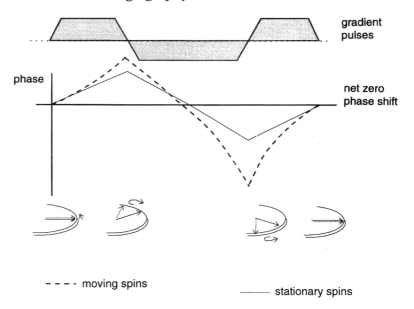

Figure 7.8. Gradient motion rephasing.

sated by simple gradient moment nulling methods. It has been shown that using reduced echo times with velocity compensation alone provides better images, than are obtained when gradient compensation is used for acceleration, with longer echo times.

Magnetic Resonance Angiography

We have seen that the magnetic resonance signal as observed in conventional images is sensitive to flow. Although conventional MR images depict regions of blood vessels, they are not capable of serving as angiographic screening tools. For this purpose, good suppression of stationary spins is essential; projections of images of the vascular tree in adequate detail also are needed. In this section we will see how flow-induced effects of phase and magnitude can be manipulated by means of appropriate pulse sequences to characterize moving spins and selectively image vessels.

The relatively new subject of MR angiography (MRA) has led to a proliferation of specialized pulse sequences and postprocessing techniques. Most of the pulse sequences for MRA can be categorized according to the flow effect (as described earlier) that was exploited to achieve contrast. The time-of-flight (**TOF**) methods achieve flow signal enhancement by taking advantage of the slice wash-in effect described earlier. Such approaches also are referred to as M_z- magnetization methods because of differences in the M_z values (spin saturation levels) that are responsible for the contrast between flowing and stationary media. The rest of the techniques may be categorized as the spin-phase methods. The flow contrast is achieved by manipulation of the phase of the spin vectors only after flipping them onto the $x'y'$ plane.

We will now consider the mechanism underlying the TOF methods in more detail. In this technique, heavily T1-weighted gradient-echo images of the region of interest are acquired, usually with the shortest possible TR and TE values. The stationary spins will experience spin saturation and will yield less signal, and spins that are flowing into the field of view will be relatively unsaturated, yielding a strong signal. This concept is an extension of single-slice flow enhancement, discussed in the "Flow Effects" section. To enhance the signal from flowing media, flow-related losses such as intravoxel phase dispersion and spin dephasing need to be minimized. Signal losses induced by phase dispersion are minimized by using small voxels. Gradient-induced spin dephasing is minimized by incorporating GMR techniques along one or more directions. Let us examine some of the specific pulse sequence strategies used to take advantage of the TOF spin saturation effect.

The sequential-slice 2D pulse sequence is a direct application of the slice wash-in effect observed in single-slice GRE images. Consider the organ being imaged as schematized in Figure 7.9. A sequential series of short TR (<50 ms), 2D-GRE images is acquired. These images differ from conventional multislice images in one very important respect: the order of phase encoding. Unlike conventional multislice imaging, entire phase-encode lines of each slice are acquired before stepping to the next slice. This method of data acquisition offers the shortest possible TR and precludes saturation of spins moving into the slice that is being imaged. At the end of the data acquisition, projections of the bright flow signal are extracted by postprocessing, most often by means of the maximum intensity ray tracing algorithm. This sequential-slice technique works best in large vessels, when the direction of flow is perpendicular to the imaged slice. Sequential 2D-MRA is used most often in examination of the femoral and iliac arteries, aorta, and portal vein. In imaging the vessels in the thoracic region, however, motion artifacts are encountered. To circumvent this drawback, a variant of the sequential 2D method can be used. One or more slices comprising the multislice stack are acquired during each respiratory cycle. Figure 7.10 shows an example of an MRI of the portal vein acquired using the breath-hold 2D-GRE technique.

The sequential 2D method has three inherent disadvantages. First, instrumental constraints on the minimum value of slice

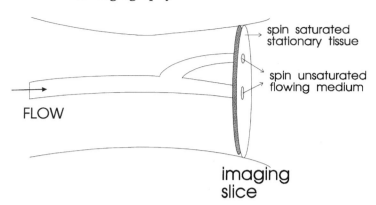

spin saturated
stationary tissue

spin unsaturated
flowing medium

FLOW

imaging
slice

Figure 7.9. 2D-MRA by imaging slices sequentially based on the concept of spin saturation of stationary spins.

thickness (>2–3 mm) yield large voxels (typically $1 \times 1 \times 5\,\text{mm}^3$), and the accompanying signal losses due to intravoxel phase dispersion can obscure small vessels. Second, nonideal slice profiles require that slices be acquired with considerable overlap, making this a rather inefficient procedure. Third, pulsating flow will appear to be somewhat saturated, causing artifactual signal loss. Despite these drawbacks, the sensitivity to slow flow has made 2D-MRA a useful MRA method. An example of the use of the sequential 2D technique is shown in Figure 7.10.

The time-of-flight volume angiography (3D-TOF) method uses a short TR/TE, 3D-GRE pulse sequence to generate images of thin contiguous slices from a thick slab of interest. The stationary spins within this slab are preferentially saturated as in the sequential 2D sequence, as a result of repeated RF excitation under very short TR (<50 ms) conditions. The flowing spins entering the

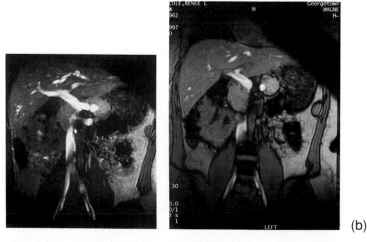

(a)   (b)

Figure 7.10. (a) Maximum intensity projection of a 2D MRA of the abdomen, reconstructed by means of multiple breath-hold coronal sections. (b) A single coronal slice comprising the image set. Courtesy of Dr. Susan Ascher.

slab during the TR period are relatively unsaturated, yielding a stronger signal. The signal from flowing spins is further enhanced by the use of GMR along the slab selection and readout directions. Just as in the 2D method, the images from the 3D partitions are processed by the maximum intensity projection algorithm to extract the angiographic projection.

There are both advantages and disadvantages to using the 3D-TOF method instead of the 2D method. The former method offers thinner slices and consequently smaller isotropic voxels, which translates to improved small vessel conspicuity. A 3D data set with isotropic voxels also yields projections at any arbitrary angle without ladder artifacts. Volume imaging is inherently less sensitive to motion artifacts because of pseudoaveraging. On the other hand, making the 3D slab thicker will produce significant saturation of the flowing medium. This imposes a practical limit on the thickness of the 3D slab for a given value of velocity.

The characteristics of 3D-TOF make it ideally suited for imaging in fast-flow applications such as the carotid and intracranial vessels. An example of the use of 3D-TOF MRA of the circle of Willis is shown in Figure 7.11. To realize the maximum enhance-

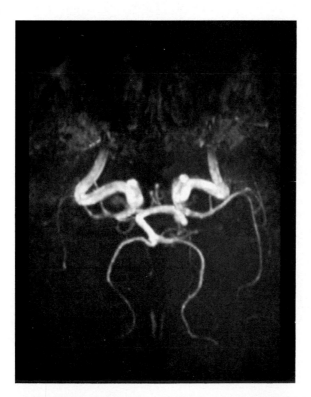

Figure 7.11. Maximum intensity projection of a brain MRA acquired by means of the 3D-TOF technique. Note appearance of periorbital structures in addition to blood vessels, made possible by short T1 of fatty tissue.

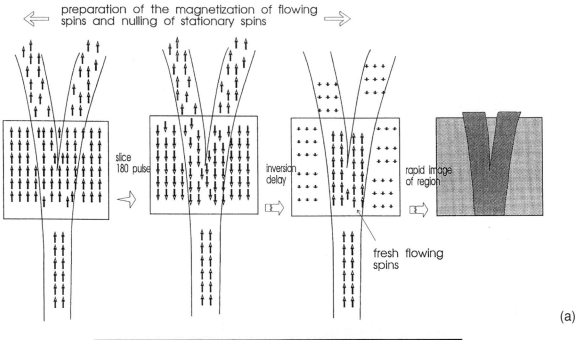

preparation of the magnetization of flowing
spins and nulling of stationary spins

slice
180 pulse

inversion
delay

rapid image
of region

fresh flowing
spins

(a)

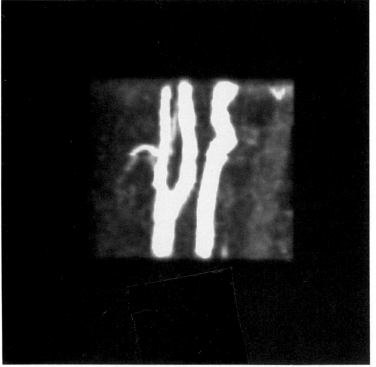

(b)

Figure 7.12. The inversion recovery MRA method: (a) schematic and (b) image (b) a carotid acquired by means of this
method.

ment of flow signal using this method, however, the RF coil must be properly chosen. If the direction of flow is along the direction of the readout or phase-encode axis, a transmit–receive coil comparable in size to the FOV should be used. Using a large transmitter coil, such as the body coil, will lead to presaturation of the flowing spins entering the FOV. Awareness of this result is particularly important for imaging of the carotids with the neck coil, since most commercially available neck coils are of the receive-only type. In these instances, sagittal and coronal slab selection will lead to presaturation of arterial blood. The implementation of axial slab selection in conjunction with readout along the z axis will give maximum flow signal.

Saturation of stationary spins can also be achieved by means of an inversion recovery (IR) approach (Figure 7.12). Here, a 180° RF pulse is applied followed by a delay period corresponding to the zero crossing time. This is similar to IR fat suppression techniques. During the inversion period, the unsaturated flowing spins populate the region within the FOV. Sampling of the moving spins at this time by rapid-scan GRE methods generates high quality MRAs. This output mode allows the use of one IR preparation for several lines of phase-encoded data, thus significantly shortening scan times. The FOV afforded by this technique is limited, however. Also, stationary components with very long or short T1 values (e.g., thrombus, cyst) can contribute to the echo. Although adding inversion recovery to sequential 2D scans will improve flow contrast, this approach is not practical because it entails increased scan times. This method has found use primarily in imaging of the carotid arteries.

The phase contrast MRA methods are based on the differences of the phase properties of moving and stationary spins. As described in the "Flow Effects" section, moving spins experience a net phase shift, while evolving in the presence of a bipolar gradient pulse. These velocity-dependent phase shifts are exploited to derive flow contrast. One of the chief advantages of this approach is that flowing spins can be differentiated from stationary spins, irrespective of their T1 values. Two scans are recorded, usually in an interleaved manner, the two acquisitions differing in the phase shifts of the flowing spins. (The unaffected stationary signal is subtracted out.) Subtraction of flow signals that have been shifted in phase to different extents yields a finite flow signal. As with TOF methods, the spin-phase techniques can be readily implemented in the 2D or 3D mode. We will now examine two specific types of pulse sequence procedure comprising this category.

The pulse sequence used in 2D phase contrast angiography is shown in Figure 7.13. In this method a bipolar gradient pulse

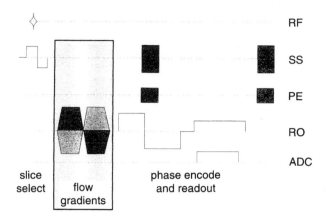

Figure 7.13. Pulse sequence for phase contrast MRA. Bipolar gradient waveforms are inserted during the echo period within a standard GRE sequence to achieve selective alteration of the phase of medium flowing along the readout direction. The sequence is repeated with opposite polarity of the bipolar gradient pair.

pair is added to the conventional GRE sequence. These gradients are independent of those used for phase-encoding and readout and lie along the direction of flow. As we saw earlier, the effect of introducing the bipolar pair will be to produce a phase shift of the flowing spins, relative to the stationary signal, given by:

$$\phi = \gamma G_v \tau T$$

where ϕ is the accumulated phase shift, τ is the width of each of the bipolar pulse, G is the value of the first gradient pulse, T is the interval between the center of the two pulses, and v is the velocity of the flowing spins. The sign of the phase shift will depend on, among other factors, the sign order of the bipolar pair. In other words, a +− pair will generate a shift opposite to that of a −+ shift (Figure 7.7). Subtraction of the raw data (echo signal) resulting from the use of bipolar pulses of opposite polarity will eliminate the signal from stationary spins. Moving spins having experienced opposite phase shifts will yield a finite signal upon subtraction.

For this method to be successful, the acquisition of echoes from opposite bipolar pulses should be interleaved to minimize motion-related artifacts. Also, the eddy currents generated from gradient switching should be negligibly small, since eddy currents themselves cause phase shifts in both moving and stationary spins. Phase shifts so produced will lead to improper subtraction of the stationary spins. When phase shifts exceed 90°, signal loss could occur because of phase aliasing (refer to the next section on velocity mapping). On the other hand, the small phase shifts from slow flow should be maximized by using strong gradients to obtain better flow signal. These two conflicting constraints limit the range of velocities observable. Also of concern is the range of velocities present during the cardiac cycle. To sample a narrower range of velocities, ECG triggering could be employed.

Several differences exist in the 2D and 3D implementations of phase contrast MRA. In the 2D implementation, the signal is acquired from a rather thick slab. This leads to noncubical voxels. Spurious signal losses can result from overlapping arterial and venous structures, andx from B_0 field inhomogeneities present across the slab. Also, the large amount of stationary spins can cause dynamic range problems. These problems are circumvented by using the 3D mode, which has provided excellent results despite the need for long scan times. Smart-encoding schemes of the bipolar gradients have been introduced recently, with a 33% saving in imaging time. Figure 7.14 shows a brain MR angiogram made by means of the 3D phase contrast technique.

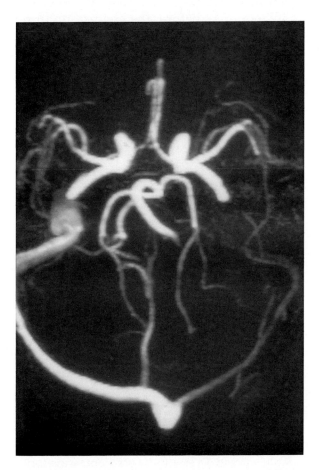

Figure 7.14. An MRA of intracranial vessels, acquired by means of the phase contrast method, with a velocity exceeding 30 cm/s. Note slow moving venous blood and absence of stationary tissue.

The magnitude contrast rephase–dephase method is another technique that exploits the phase effects of moving spins. The pulse sequence used in this approach is shown in Figure 7.15. Just as in the phase contrast method, each phase-encode line is acquired twice, first with gradient moment·nulling (flow compensation) and then without gradient moment nulling. The flow-compensated gradient pulses is applied parallel to the direction of flow. Unlike the preceding method, however, the raw data are not subtracted. The image reconstructed from the flow-compensated echo (rephase image) is subtracted from that obtained without flow compensation (dephase image). Spins that were flowing along the direction of the rephase–dephase gradient will be affected differently in the two images, but the stationary medium will be of equal intensity in both. Therefore subtraction of the dephase image from the rephase image will eliminate the stationary signal, yielding an angiographic image.

As with the phase contrast, this pulse sequence is most often used in the 3D mode. As before, the acquisition of rephase and dephase data is interleaved to minimize misregistration effects. The flow signal attainable using this technique is largely deter-

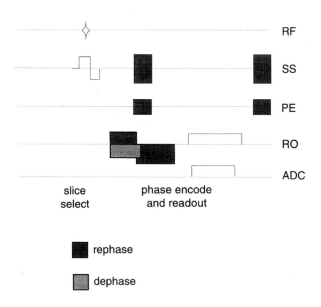

Figure 7.15. Pulse sequence for magnitude contrast (also known as rephase–dephase) MRA. Readout gradient waveform alternated between flow-compensated (rephase) and non-flow-compensated (dephase) modes. The magnitude images are subtracted to get the MRA image.

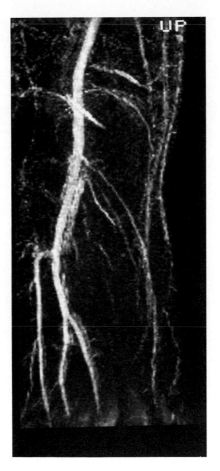

Figure 7.16. An MRA of the popliteal vessels, acquired by subtraction of flow rephase and dephase images.

mined by the extent of flow dephasing achieved in the dephase image. This in turn is governed by the flow velocity and by the magnitude of the readout gradients. Because of practical constraints associated with the latter, this technique works best with flow velocities above 10 cm/s. The use of the readout gradients for dephasing the spins precludes combining flow data from other directions because this would necessitate repeating the scan with different frequency-encode directions. Because of the foregoing constraints, this technique has found use mostly for imaging the vessels of the femoral–popliteal system. Figure 7.16 presents an example of a popliteal MRA.

With the recent technological improvements in MRI instrumentation, rapid high resolution scanning has opened the way for the use of contrast agents in MRA. The use of contrast agents for MRA is a concept borrowed from X-ray angiography, which is often considered as the diagnostic gold standard. In this

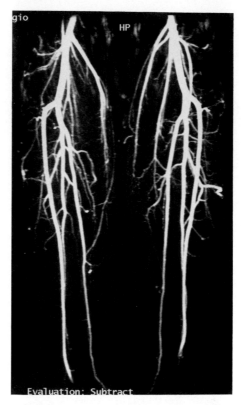

Figure 7.17. An MRA of the lower extremities, acquired by subtracting precontrast from postcontrast rapid gradient echo images.

approach, two sets of images are acquired rapidly, one before and another after injection of contrast agent. The contrast agent present in the vessels causes an increase in the vascular signal due to T1 shortening. Pixel-wise subtraction of the precontrast from the postcontrast images results in MRA images. In many instance just post-contrast images will suffice. Although only a limited FOV can be imaged in the small time interval afforded by the vascular phase of the contrast agent, excellent MRAs of the major vessels as well the lower extremities can in fact be recorded a very short scan period. An example of popliteal branches imaged by means of this subtraction angiography appears in Figure 7.17.

The clinical efficacy of MRA in general has been slow to be accepted. However, carotid and intracranial vessel MR angiograms have become well-accepted screening tools. As long as the techniques themselves are rapidly improving, it will be difficult to demonstrate efficacy in studies with large numbers of patients. The distinct advantage of being able to record true 3D information using MRA assures this technique a place in the radiologist's tool chest for the near future.

Velocity Mapping

As we have seen, magnetic resonance can be used to image flow in vessels. This flow sensitivity of the MR signal can be used to quantitate flow, and to measure velocities during the various phases of the cardiac cycle. Publications citing the ability of MR to assess flow appeared as early as 1956, well preceding reports of imaging applications. As with MRA, both magnitude and phase components of the magnetization have been used to measure flow. Since the blood flow in the vessels is pulsatile, these measurements are best made in conjunction with ECG gating. Among the various magnitude techniques that have gained wide acceptance are the bolus-tracking, and zebra stripe, methods.

In the bolus-tracking technique, the simplest method, flow is measured by observing the propagation of a saturation band applied to the moving blood. Interestingly, blood flow measurement in the body by means of, tagging or bolus tracking, historically preceded MR imaging. However, the results were accomplished with continuous wave NMR rather than pulsed NMR, as used in MRI instruments.

The pulse sequence used in bolus tagging is shown in Figure 7.18. This method applies a gradient-echo technique to image a slice parallel to the flow direction. The flowing spins are tagged by applying a presaturation band perpendicular to the direction of flow: an additional slice selection pulse corresponding to the saturation band is inserted for every phase-encode line in the pulse sequence. The delay period (generally 10–100 ms) between the saturation pulse and the imaging slice selection pulse (flow

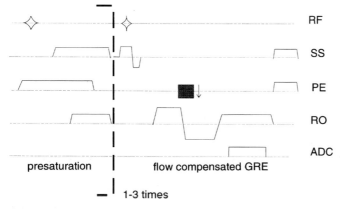

Figure 7.18. The pulse sequence used for bolus-tagging velocity quantification.

delay) causes the saturated region to shift in position relative to the rest of the saturated band. Velocities are then computed from the measurement of the ratio of the displacement of the saturated band to the delay period.

One of the chief advantages of this method is the ease of implementation of the pulse sequence. If the slice thickness is greater than the lumen size of the vessel, the resulting partial volume artifact can obscure the propagation of the bolus. As the bolus propagates, the z magnetization of the bolus recovers as a function of its T1 time. When the delay period extends to a value four times T1, it has lost most of the difference in z magnetization. If the T1 recovery is complete during the flow delay period, the tagged region will be isointense with the untagged region, making it difficult to identify the moving saturation band. Because of this effect of T1, bolus tagging should be performed before the administration of contrast agents. Although ECG gating is necessary for quantitative measurements, the breath-hold GRE sequences can be used for qualitative studies. Bolus tagging is well suited for differentiating a true from a false lumen in aortic dissections and in evaluating portal venous flow. Normal portal flow can be demonstrated by means of this method, as indicated in Figure 7.19.

A continuous wave (CW) NMR method has been successfully used in some instruments. In this approach a steady source of radio frequency supplies the irradiation, instead of a pulsed source, and the NMR signal is detected by varying the static

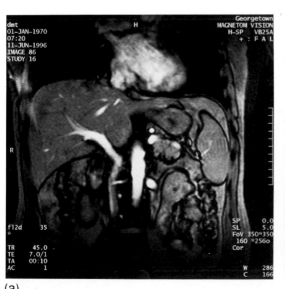
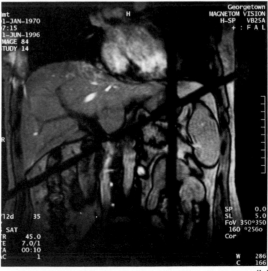

(a)   (b)

Figure 7.19. Normal portal flow demonstrated by means of a bolus-tracking pulse (a) without saturation and (b) with saturation. Note loss of portal vein signal and shift in the edge of the saturation band.

magnetic field. In the application of CW NMR for flow measurement, the flowing blood is irradiated continuously upstream. The detector coil placed downstream detects the NMR signal emitted by the blood as it flows by. The amplitude of the detected signal is a function of the velocity of flow and the T1 relaxation time of blood. The signal increases with increase in velocity of flow. Calibration of the flow signal by means of a phantom permits the computation of flow rates. Although this technique provides real-time measurements of flow rates, no spatial information is present. The detected signal arises from the whole region under the receiver coil rather from than a specific vessel.

In addition to the magnitude (M_z) based methods discribed in the previous section, phase shift based techniques can also be used for velocity measurement. The direct relationship between phase shifts and velocity allows precise measurement of velocity by mapping the phase shifts in the image.

The phase-sensitive receiver of an MRI instrument acquires the two components for each pixel: $a \sin\phi$ and $a \cos\phi$. The two components are generally referred to as the real and imaginary components. Conventional MR images display only the magnitude a (absolute value) of the complex pair. The absolute value is computed pixel-wise according to equation 7.5.

$$a = \left[(a\sin\phi)^2 + (a\cos\phi)^2 \right]^{1/2} \qquad (7.5)$$

The phase information corresponding to the orientation of the vector in the x-y plane is not present in these images. This phase angle ϕ may be computed pixel-wise from the arctangent of the ratio of real to imaginary data as shown in equation 7.6.

$$\phi = \arctan\left[\frac{a\sin\phi}{a\cos\phi} \right] \qquad (7.6)$$

In this mode of data display, pixels with zero phase shifts will appear gray, and pixels with positive and negative phase shifts will appear brighter and darker, respectively. Although this method is readily implemented, the phase data are easily obscured by spurious phase shifts. Other sources of phase shifts include patient motion and eddy currents. In GRE sequences B_0 heterogeneity and chemical shifts can contribute to the net phase shift displayed by the pixel. For the reasons just cited, this method is best used with spin-echo sequences when detecting small phase shifts. Since spin-echo sequences are insensitive to B_0 inhomogeneities, the primary difficulty with the implementation of phase mapping is one of aliasing. Aliasing can manifest itself in two ways. The first has to do with the periodic nature of the phase shift. Any phase shift that is $360 + \phi$ will appear as ϕ, as

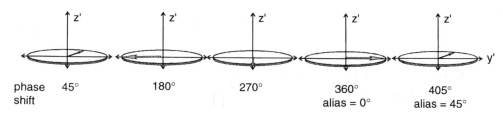

phase   45°   180°   270°   360°   405°
shift   alias = 0°   alias = 45°

Figure 7.20. When phase shift exceeds 360° aliasing occurs. Increase in phase is demonstrated from left to right.

shown in Figure 7.20. The two vectors with phase shifts of 360 + ϕ and ϕ are positioned the same.

The second type of phase aliasing is inherent in the computation of phase angle using the inverse tangent function. This effect can be understood by examining the plot of $\tan\phi$ versus ϕ shown in Figure 7.21.

When ϕ is greater than 90° or less than −90°, some ambiguities are noted. The value of $\tan(90 + \phi)$ is equal to $\tan - (90 - \phi)$ and that of $\tan(90 - \phi)$ is equal to $\tan - (90 + \phi)$. Thus pixels with a phase shift of 120° will have the same intensity as those with a phase shift of −60°. This implies that spins moving in one direction, fast enough to accrue a phase shift exceeding 90°, will undergo aliasing.

In practice, the phase shifts are precisely calibrated, using flow phantoms to determine the upper limit of the velocity that can be detected without aliasing.

Despite the drawback of the aliasing effects, phase contrast imaging has been routinely used for flow estimation. A rapid

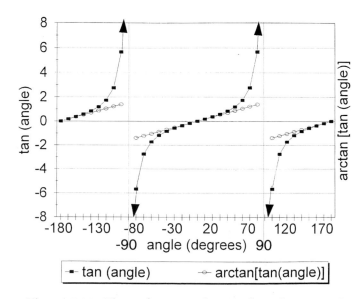

Figure 7.21. Plots of $\tan\phi$ and $\arctan[\tan\phi]$ versus ϕ].

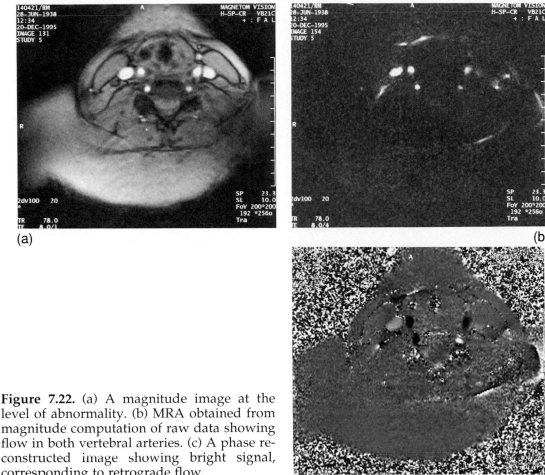

Figure 7.22. (a) A magnitude image at the level of abnormality. (b) MRA obtained from magnitude computation of raw data showing flow in both vertebral arteries. (c) A phase reconstructed image showing bright signal, corresponding to retrograde flow.

GRE pulse sequence with bipolar gradients is used to generate the phase shift in the flowing spins. Figure 7.13 showed the pulse sequence timing of a GRE sequence with flow sensitization along the slice-select direction. If the echo is recorded in synchronization with the cardiac cycle, a velocity profile during the entire cardiac cycle can be obtained. The use of ECG-synchronized phase mapping is demonstrated in Figure 7.22 in a patient. Carotid TOF MRA demonstrated abnormal flow signal in the left vertebral artery. Phase contrast images at the location of the abnormality indicated retrograde flow during some parts of the cardiac cycle.

Another implementation of the phase mapping technique is the zebra stripe method, in which a linear phase change is deliberately introduced along the readout axis (flow direction). This is easily accomplished by acquiring off-centered echoes. The linear phase shift will cause a periodic variation of signal along the readout direction. Any flow-induced phase shift will add to this

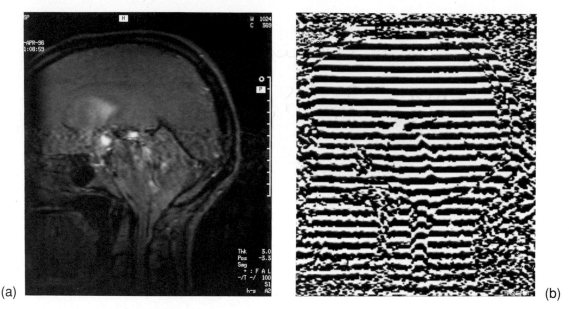

Figure 7.23. Zebra stripe motion imaging of the spinal cord: (a) magnitude images and (b) zebra stripe real-valued image.

baseline zebra pattern and will appear as displacements in the vertical stripes, as shown in Figure 7.23. The phase shifts can be quantitatively determined by measuring the displacements of the flowing stripes relative to the baseline zebra pattern of the stationary spins. An advantage of this technique is that it does not suffer from aliasing effects.

Fourier velocity imaging, another phase shift based method, allows accurate measurement of velocity information by phase encoding velocity. In generating an anatomical image, a single gradient pulse, stepped through a series of values, is used to perform phase encoding. If a bipolar gradient waveform is used instead (Figure 7.24), only the spins moving along the gradient

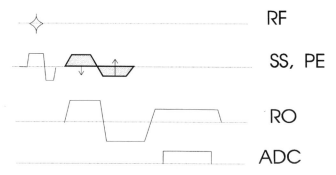

Figure 7.24. Bipolar stepped gradient pulses are used for phase encoding to selectively encode flowing spins.

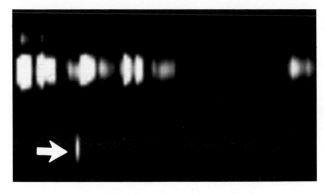

Figure 7.25. Fourier flow imaging showing displacement of the flow signal (arrow).

direction will be phase-encoded. This is because stationary spins, unlike moving spins, do not experience a net phase shift. Therefore, in the resulting image, the stationary spins will appear as a single line at the zero phase-encode position. The signals from moving spins are further dispersed above or below this line depending on the direction and velocity of flow. Typically, the direction of flow phase encoding is chosen to be the same as the slice-select direction. Therefore, only the spins flowing normal to the slice will be imaged.

As in the other methods, precise measurement of velocities requires ECG gating of every phase-encode line of data. Just as in phase encoding of stationary spins, flow encoding is susceptible to wraparound effects (aliasing) and therefore requires properly chosen gradient amplitudes. The relative excess of stationary spins over flowing spins will cause dynamic range problems and therefore calls for some form of attenuation of stationary spin signal (presaturation). Another disadvantage is the lack of anatomical information, necessitating a localizer image for establishing anatomical landmarks. On the other hand, this method offers excellent temporal and spatial resolution, allowing flow quantification. The flow in the popliteal vessel across a slice located at the knee level is shown in Figure 7.25. In this example, the flow in the popliteal artery appears as a displaced blip whereas the veinous flow is not visible because of presaturation.

Additional Reading

Anderson CM, Edelman RR, Turski PA. Clinical magnetic resonance Angiography. New York: Raven Press, 1993.
Potchen EJ, Haocke EM, Siebert JE, Gottschalk A. Magnetic resonance Angiography: Concepts and applications.
Chicago: Mosby-Year Book, 1993.

8

Spectroscopy

nuclei =
$H^1, P^{31}, C^{13}, Na^{23}$

In magnetic resonance imaging, the nuclear magnetic resonance effect is exploited to give signal intensity distribution as a function of spatial coordinates, as dictated by the Larmor equation. The signal intensities are further modified by the inherent differences in tissue properties such as T1 and T2. In addition, only signal from water and fat is observed, since relatively high concentrations of these protons are present in tissue. The NMR resonance phenomenon can also be used to yield information on chemical structure and composition. This is the basis for NMR spectroscopy, which by definition is the study of the intensity patterns of NMR signal as a function of spectral frequency.

Historically, NMR spectroscopy preceded imaging by several decades and is now routinely used by organic chemists as an analytical tool. In the simplest terms, an observation of two resonances (e.g., of water and of fat) in routine imaging is a spectroscopic effect. Spectroscopy is relevant in the human because it has the potential for noninvasively acquiring metabolic information from tissue. As a diagnostic tool, it could provide information complementary to that of MR imaging in much the same manner as position emission tomography (PET) imaging. Most of the instrumentation used in imaging is also used in spectroscopy. However, the spectroscopy data usually are presented in a plot format (spectrum) and less often as a metabolite map such as in PET images.

Before we examine the exact mechanism for the origin of the spectroscopic effect, it will help to understand the scope of NMR spectroscopy in biology. The technique of spectroscopy is capable of detecting millimolar concentrations of certain metabolites that have paramagnetic nuclei. Some relevant nuclei are ^{1}H, ^{31}P, ^{13}C, and ^{23}Na. To be detectable, the molecules must also be small enough to enable free rotation in the time scale of spin relaxation. Some molecules that fall in this category are water, lactate, glucose, and high energy phosphates. The ability to detect these compounds directly in vivo is of paramount importance in answering questions relating to tissue metabolism. It should be noted that large molecules such as proteins and small substrates bound to large molecules are not easily studied by means of in vivo spectroscopy.

To understand how chemical species can be differentiated by NMR techniques, we revisit the Larmor equation, according to which the resonance frequency is proportional to the magnitude of the static field, where the proportionality factor is the gyromagnetic ratio. At the outset, no attempt was made to differentiate the magnetic field experienced by the nuclei (B_e) from that applied by the magnet (B_0). In reality, B_e is not the same as B_0, except for a isolated nucleus. This is because the nucleus is surrounded by the negatively charged electron cloud, which interacts with B_0. The Larmor equation for molecules needs to be rewritten to include the effects of the electron interaction as follows:

$$h\nu = \gamma B_e = \gamma(B_0 - \sigma B_0) \tag{8.1}$$

where σ is a corrective factor, known as the shielding factor. The electron cloud thus exerts a shielding influence, and the magnetic field at the nucleus is less than that applied by the magnet. In addition, the reduction in the magnetic field due to the electron cloud is directly proportional to the applied static field. The shielding factors σ will depend on several factors, the most significant being the electronic structure of the molecule. Other factors that will alter the shielding factor are temperature and chemical exchange phenomena. Typically the shielding factor will decrease the resonance frequencies by a minute extent, generally by 10^{-6} to 10^{-4} (1 ppm to 100 ppm) of the Larmor frequency.

The shielding factor σ is exquisitely sensitive to the local electronic environment, and thus molecular moieties that are even slightly different will resonate at different frequencies. For example, the molecule ethanol, which contains three methyl protons, two methylene protons, and one hydroxy proton, will exhibit three different Larmor frequencies. This is because the magnetic environment of these three groups of protons are slightly different, despite being from the same molecule. Since these frequency differences result from chemical structure, they are referred to as chemical shifts (δ). These three distinct resonances may be observed by Fourier analysis of the FID resulting from a nonselective RF pulse. In addition, the intensities of the three resonances will reflect the number of each kind of proton. Such a plot of intensity versus chemical shift is known as a spectrum (Figure 8.1).

The chemical shift is generally expressed in units of parts per million (ppm) of the unshifted Larmor frequency:

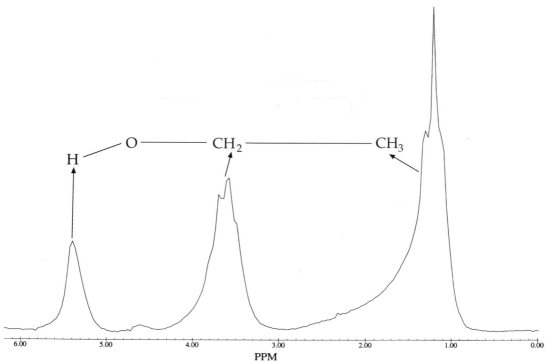

Figure 8.1. The three resonances from ethanol.

$$\delta = \frac{\omega_e - \omega_0}{10^{-6}\omega_0} \; ppm \tag{8.2}$$

where w_0 is the unshifted and w_e the shifted Larmor frequencies.

For example, the Larmor frequency at a static field of 1.5 T is 63 MHz (63×10^6 Hz); 1 ppm of the Larmor frequency is therefore 63 Hz ($63 \times 10^6 \times 10^{-6}$ Hz). The methyl and methylene resonances are separated by 0.5 ppm, which is equal to 31.5 Hz. If the sample were studied at a field of 4.7 T, the frequency shift would be 100 Hz, which translates of 0.5 ppm. Although the absolute resonance frequencies will be different at different static fields of a given proton, the chemical shift will always be the same for all static fields. Since it is impossible to measure the unshifted frequency of a naked nucleus, the chemical shift of a reference molecule is arbitrarily set to zero and the shifts of all other resonances are expressed relative to the reference standard. For protons and carbon, this reference is tetramethyl silane (TMS); for phosphorus, the shift is relative to phosphocreatine (or sometimes phosphoric acid). The NMR spectrum of every molecule thus displays a characteristic pattern, with a unique combination of peak positions and intensities. This is why spectroscopy will aid in structure determination or, conversely, in the measurement of concentrations (or ratios of concentrations) of metabolites. Table 8.1 lists the chemical shifts of common metabolites.

A uniform static field B_0, over the volume of interest, is crucial for recording NMR spectra. Magnetic field inhomogeneity will cause the different parts of the sample to have different Larmor frequencies for the chemical species. The different Larmor frequencies will result in broadened spectral lines. Line broadening induced by B_0 field inhomogeneity can obscure chemical shifts and therefore needs to be minimized. The process of optimizing the field uniformity, or "shimming", usually precedes all spectroscopy studies. It is performed by adjusting the electric currents in the individual channels of the shim coils. In one common approach, the currents are adjusted by iteration, to maximize the water FID signal. The FID signal recorded from a sample in a inhomogeneous field will decay faster than one in a uniform field. This is due to phase dispersion effects (also called the T2* effect). Figure 8.2 shows an example of an FID and spectrum before and after shimming.

Just as in imaging, the relaxation properties T1 and T2 will greatly affect the appearance of spectra. The amplitude of a recorded spectrum will be attenuated if the RF pulse repetition time TR is less than T1 × 5. This effect is equivalent to that of T1 weighting observed in imaging upon decreasing the value of TR. Unlike data for imaging, spectroscopy data usually are acquired under fully relaxed conditions. This is done by the combined use of small flip angles and long TR. In some instances the spectroscopy data are acquired using short TR, and known values of T1 weighting (saturation factors) are used in the computation of the fully relaxed amplitude.

Table 8.1. Chemical Shifts, δ for Some Common Metabolites

Proton[a]	δ (ppm)	Phosphorus[b]	δ (ppm)	Carbon[a]	δ (ppm)
Water	4.76	γ-ATP	−2.38	Glucose C1	92.7
Lipid	1.2	β-ATP	−16	Glycogen C1	100.5
Lactate	1.3	α-ATP	−7.45		
Creatine	3	Phosphocreatine (PCR)			
Choline	3.2	Inorganic phosphate (Pi)	4.88		
N-Acetylospartate	2	Phospho diesters (PDE)	2.9		
Silione	−0.5	Phospho mono esters (PME)	6.64		

[a] TMS is reference.
[b] Phosphocreatine is reference.

NMR1™

Seconds

(a)

NMR1™

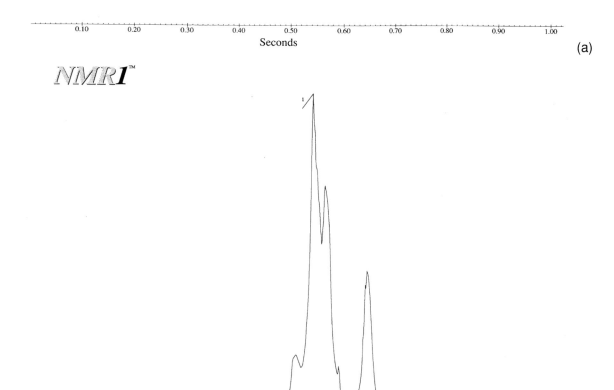

PPM

(b)

Figure 8.2. FID (a) and spectrum (b) before and after (c,d) shimming. Note longer decay times and narrower spectral peaks for shimmed data.

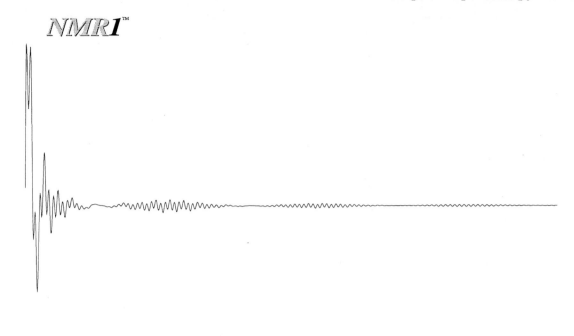

(c)

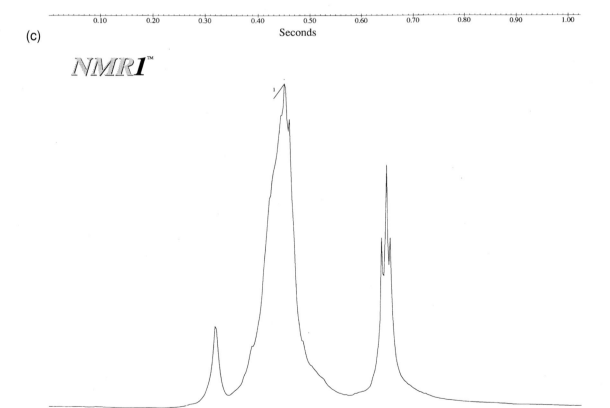

(d)

Figure 8.2. *Continued*

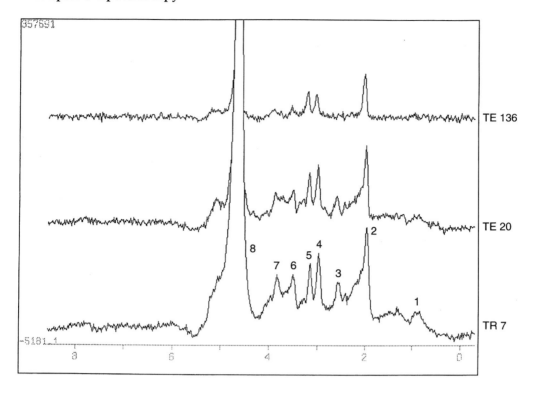

Figure 8.3. Volume-localized, water-suppressed spectra acquired from normal brain at three different echo times (7, 20, 136 ms). Peak assignments: 1, lipids; 2, *N*-acetylaspartate; 3, glutamine and glutamate; 4, creatine and phosphcreatine; 5, choline; 6, myoinositol; 7, creatine; 8, residual water resonance. (Courtesy of Stefan Posse, National Institutes of Health.)

The effect of spin relaxation time T2 is manifest in T2-weighted spin-echo images as diminished signal from components possessing short T2 values. The same effect is observed in certain echo-based spectroscopy techniques, where the intensity of the peaks is influenced by the echo time used in the pulse sequence. Figure 8.3 shows two spectra recorded from a region in the brain with three different echo times: 7, 20, and 136 ms. Note the decreased signal in the spectra with longer TE. In addition to the intensity changes, the T2 values will determine the natural line widths of the peaks. The natural line width is inversely proportional to the T2 relaxation time. However, the line widths of peaks in spectra recorded in vivo are generally limited by the B_0 inhomogeneity (T2* effect).

Scalar coupling is a phenomenon that is responsible for the splitting of peaks noted in high resolution NMR spectra and has no parallel in routine MRI. The spectrum in Figure 8.2d (aqueous ethanol) was recorded under well-shimmed conditions (<5 Hz). The broad resonances, present in Figure 8.2a, had been resolved

further into multiplets. To understand this effect, referred to as
spin–spin splitting, consider the B_e experienced by the protons
on the methyl group. As explained earlier, the effective field is
influenced by the applied static field and the induced shielding
field, which is responsible for chemical shifts. In addition, the
effective field is modified by the spin state of the neighboring
protons. Let us consider a two-proton spin system (A–B), connected by a network of chemical bonds, as shown in Figure 8.4.

The NMR resonance arises from the spin energy levels of each
of the protons, as determined by the orientation of the spin
vector relative to the direction of B_0. Since the protons act like
magnetic dipoles, the B_e of proton A will also depend on the
relative orientation of proton B, and vice versa. This orientation
dependence is transmitted through the electronic clouds comprising the molecular bonds. While in the absence of proton B, a
single resonance frequency is observed (from two energy states),
the presence of proton B generates four energy states. The same
effect occurs for proton B because of the orientation dependence

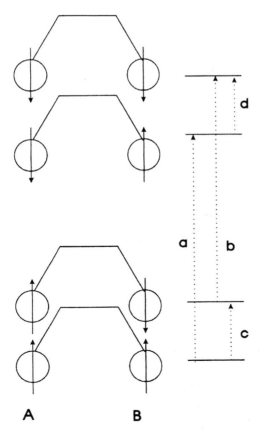

Figure 8.4. The four resonances that arise from spin–spin coupling of
two nuclei, A and B.

of proton A. Thus each resonance is split into a pair of resonances a,b and c,d. If the chemical shift of the two protons is different, a total of four spectral peaks will be observed.

The splitting of the resonances will further depend on the number of protons coupled. In general, a coupling with n equivalent protons will give rise to $n + 1$ multiplets. Thus, in the case of ethanol, the protons of the methyl group having the same chemical shift are split into three peaks by the two methylene protons. Similarly, the methylene protons are split into four peaks by the three methyl protons. In addition, a proton can be coupled to more than one set of protons, which can generate further splitting of the resonance. Clearly, the appearance of the spectral multiplet structure is exquisitely sensitive to changes in molecular structure. Thus the study of splitting patterns can aid in molecular structure determination of unknown compounds.

The splitting of the resonances due to spin coupling is typically of the order of 1–10 Hz. Also, in contrast to the chemical shift effect, which is linearly dependent on the static magnetic field, scalar coupling is independent of the magnitude of the static magnetic field. The extent of the splitting (referred to as J-coupling) also depends on other factors, such as the chemical shift difference of the two resonances and the molecular orientation.

Molecular Exchange

The appearance of spectra can be altered by dynamic chemical processes, such as molecular exchange reactions, that occur during NMR data acquisition. Both the line width and the chemical shift of the observed lines are affected by chemical exchange processes involving the protons responsible for the resonances. This effect is particularly relevant in biological systems, where protons are in a constant state of chemical exchange. For example, protons bonded to bulk water molecules are constantly exchanging with water molecules bound to macromolecules. Consider the case of a proton (H^+ ion) hopping between two environments, A and B. Further assume that the chemical shift of the proton differs at these two environments (δ_1 and δ_2). If the proton exchange process is frozen for a relatively long time, two distinct NMR resonances will be observed at chemical shifts δ_1 and δ_2. If, however, the exchange process occurs faster than the difference in the Larmor precessional frequencies at those two sites, only a single resonance frequency will be detected. This frequency will be the weighted mean of the resonances in the absence of exchange.

Two particular cases of molecular exchange are particularly relevant to magnetic resonance of biological systems. The first is the exchange reaction of the water molecules present in tissue. The water molecules in tissue are continously hopping between two environments. The first is bulk water, with a narrow resonance. The second is the bound state with macromolecules, which yield a rather broad resonance, several kilohertz wide (Figure 8.5).

The exchange rate is slow with respect to the NMR time scale and thus yields two resonances. The broad component is not usually detected because of its extremely short spin–spin relaxation time. This exchange process is exploited for generating magnetization/transfer image contrast. In this technique, the intensity of water protons engaged in slow exchange is suppressed by off-resonance irradiation intense enough to saturate the broad components. Some of the saturated water molecules end up in the other pool as a result of the exchange process. Upon detecting the narrow resonant component, the saturated water protons contribute to the diminution of signal.

The second case of exchange of importance to biological systems has to do with the acid–base equilibrium of aqueous orthophosphoric acid, which is present in tissue and represented in equation 8.3.

$$H_2PO_4^- \rightleftharpoons HPO_4^{2-} + H^+ \tag{8.3}$$

The exchange rate is fast compared to the difference in chemical shifts, and therefore only one exchange-narrowed resonance is observed by phosphorus NMR spectroscopy. Furthermore, reactive changes in the concentration of the cations will cause any change in pH to shift the frequency of resonance. For example, an increase in the pH will lead to an increased reverse reaction, which will move the weighted mean chemical shift of the two phosphorus nuclei. Therefore the chemical shift of the inorganic phosphate in tissue is a sensitive indicator of tissue pH and can be used to noninvasively determine tissue pH.

NMR spectroscopy can yield invaluable metabolic information, but only if spectroscopic data can be recorded from a selective region of the tissue. For example, one might ask how the spectrum from a cancerous region of tissue differs from a region

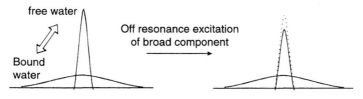

Figure 8.5. Spectra of free and bound water: magnetization transfer between the two components exchanging water leads to drop in the detected signal of the free water.

of normal brain matter. Clearly a precise control of the region of interest is desirable, since a spectrum of the whole head region will not provide the specific information. The need for spectroscopic information from specific volume elements within the imaging field has spawned a new area of study called **in vivo** localized volume spectroscopy.

At the outset, two different strategies may be considered to selectively record volume data. In the first approach only a selective volume element is excited by the RF pulses. This will result in data from the chosen region only. The alternate approach is to record data within the whole volume of the RF coil and subsequently resolve the components corresponding to the various spatial regions. In practice, a combination of these methods has been found to be more useful rather than relying on one or the other. As an example of the first approach, we may cite a surface coil employed to limit the region of tissue under observation. Further localization may be achieved by performing slice-selective excitations. As an example of the second approach, we mention phase-encoding gradients used along one or more directions to generate spatial maps of the spectral resonances. The sections that follow describe a few specific spectroscopy techniques.

The simplest localization method, both technically and conceptually, is the use of a local coil for RF excitation and reception. Since the sensitive volume of the coil will only extend as deep as the radius of the coil, all outlying tissue will not contribute to the signal (and the noise!). Thus limited localization is achieved along one axis, that normal to the plane of the surface coil. When a surface coil is used, however, the flip angle experienced by the spin system is not constant but a function of the coil design and

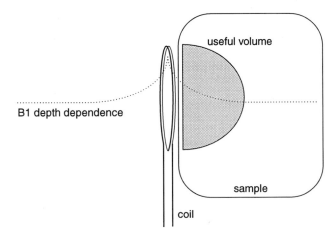

Figure 8.6. Surface coil volume localization, showing depth dependence of signal.

Adiabatic RF Pulses   When a rectangular RF pulse is used for excitation, the flip angle is B_1 field dependent and varies according to Figure 8.6. An adiabatic RF pulse permits a constant flip angle, independent of B_1 variation across the sample. This is performed by carrying out the analogue of the adiabatic half-passage experiment. The sensitivity of the coil still falls off nonlinearly from the coil, since signal reception sensitivity is a function of distance. The adiabatic pulse provides an improvement in SNR due to absence of signal cancellation stemming from out-of-phase signal as in the case of rectangular pulse. Adiabatic pulses can also be used to generate spin-echo images, using a surface coil. This is not possible using rectangular pulses because a uniform 90 and 180° flip angle cannot be achieved across the sample.

size. This disadvantage is schematically described in Figure 8.6 for a surface coil; the shaded region indicates the accessible region of sample. The dotted line approximates the falloff in B_1 as a function of depth.

The localization achieved with a surface coil may be further improved upon in a number of ways. The simplest method of further limiting the sensitive volume to deeper tissue is achieved by manipulation of the RF power and phase. One such method, known as the depth pulse **sequence**, uses a train of 90° and 180° RF pulses with suitable combinations of RF phase to select out a region of sample experiencing a narrow range of flip angles.

The underlying principle can be gleaned by examining the effect of the following RF preparation. Consider the effect of a pair of RF pulses, the second twice as great in amplitude as the first, followed in due course by FID acquisition. The sequence is repeated four times, where the phase of the second RF pulse is incremented by 90°. The receiver phase is alternated for every other acquisition. Only regions experiencing a flip combination of 90° and 180° will yield the maximum signal.

The reason for this can be understood by examining the spin vectors as a result of the two RF excitations. Figure 8.7 compares the vectorial changes for two regions under the coil that experience flip angles 30 and 90°. For the sake of simplicity, let us consider the effect of two RF repetitions instead of four and examine the position of the vector after each pulse pair. The top row in Figure 8.7 shows the changes for the isochromats with a flip angle of 30° and the bottom row for 90°. The net signal is the vectorial sum of the vectors from each RF pulse pair. For the 90° flip angle, maximum signal is generated because both excitations generate vectors that are collinear. For the 30° flip angle, how-

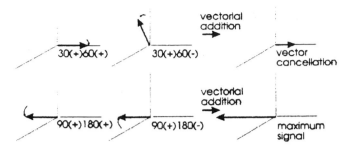

Figure 8.7. Localization of regions using pairs of RF pulses with a surface coil: effects for deeper tissue (top) and for tissue closer to the coil (bottom).

ever, the two vectors are not collinear and the vectorial sum is less than the case of 90° flip angle. It can be seen that even a simple scheme such as this one will lead to enhancement of signal from regions experiencing a 90° flip angle. This principle can be extended to include more RF pulses and has been successfully used to obtain spectra of the liver, without contamination of the overlying muscle tissue. It is difficult to justify its routine use in a clinical setting, however, because of the excessive RF power deposited in tissue.

Another technique, known as **rotating frame zeugmatography**, has been proposed to obtain to a 2D data set without the use of field gradient switching. An FID is recorded for a series of RF voltage values, and upon 2D Fourier transformation, a B_1 field-sensitive spectral set is obtained. Spectral information is presented along the first dimension, and the B_1 field is represented along the second dimension. Since, however, the B_1 field isocontours tend to curve back toward the plane of the coil, the spectra do not represent pure depth dependence. Nonetheless, this method has been used successfully to record localized spectra.

Just as in conventional imaging, pulsed field gradients can be used to selectively study a specific region lying within the RF coil. In the simplest case, the FID resulting from a selected slice can be collected. Conversely, the signal from a slice of tissue underlying the surface coil can be rejected, using the presaturation technique (slice excitation followed by spin dephasing). One or more slice selections can be used to select the volume region. For example, a cubical region is selected by the use of three successive 90° pulses, in conjunction with the three different gradient pulses as shown Figure 8.8. Only the region that has experienced all three RF excitations will generate a stimulated echo. The spin echoes generated in the excitation process are carefully avoided by appropriately timing the crusher gradient pulses. More recently, cylindrical regions have been selected by the concurrent use of two gradients during an RF pulse.

Although slice selection is convenient for selecting a region of study, the method is not without problems. Slice misregistration and T2 losses are the primary disadvantages. Slice misregistration is caused by signal contribution of the spectral components, which are off-resonance, but lying in a spatially shifted region. As a result, the various peaks forming the spectrum originate from slightly shifted regions, making interpretations difficult. For example, consider the case of the resonances for PME and β-ATP, separated by approximately 20 ppm (500 Hz at 1.5 T). If a gradient strength of 5 mT/m is used during slice selection, the slices corresponding to the two resonances will be separated by approximately 6 cm. All the intermediate resonances will arise from regions lying between them. To minimize this error in volume selection, the strongest gradient strength possible needs to be used. Also, for proton spectroscopy this problem is not significant because the gyromagnetic ratio is higher and the chemical shift scale is relatively compressed.

The other problem associated with performing slice selections is the spin evolution that occurs during the selection if more than one slice-select is performed. In phosphorus spectroscopy the signal loss due to T2 decay can be significant. Nevertheless, many techniques involving slice selection have been successfully implemented. The alternate approach is to use gradient pulses for phase encoding the data, just as in MR imaging. Implementation may be in one or more directions to enhance the spatial resolution. This technique is referred to as chemical shift imaging (CSI). In practice, the combined use of slice-select and phase-encode has proved to be useful.

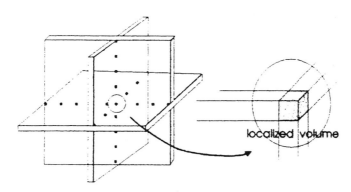

Figure 8.8. Volume selection from three slice selection preparations.

Localized Spectroscopy Methods

Depth-Resolved Surface Coil Spectroscopy (DRESS)

DRESS uses the simplest method of a single slice selection to localize the region of interest (Figure 8.9). A gradient pulse is applied concurrently with an RF pulse of limited bandwidth. The frequency of the RF pulse is shifted to excite the desired slice, and the resulting gradient echo is acquired, as an FID. A disk-shaped region of the sample lying under the coil will contribute to the signal. Figure 8.9 is a schematic diagram of the pulse sequence. This method has the advantage of yielding good resolution and short echo times. Thus, species with short T2 values may be easily detected. The DRESS method has been used to study phosphorus spectra of muscle, heart, and tumors.

Fast Rotating Gradient Spectroscopy (FROGS)

The FROGS technique (Figure 8.10) is complementary to the DRESS method just described, in that everything underlying the coil except a disk-shaped region will contribute to the signal. Implementation begins with the performance of a slice selection as described above. The resulting signal is phase-dispersed by means of gradient pulses (this step is also known as presaturation). A nonselective RF pulse is used to sample the magnetization of the rest of the sensitive volume. Because of signal reception immediately following the RF pulse, T2 decay is minimized. However, species with short T1 will recover during the spoiling period and contribute to the detected signal. This method has found use especially in recording liver spectra without contamination of overlying muscle tissue.

Image-Selected In Vivo Spectroscopy (ISIS)

The ISIS method is commonly used to record phosphorus spectra from one or more cubical regions in the brain. This pulse sequence uses a series of frequency-selective 180° pulses, in or-

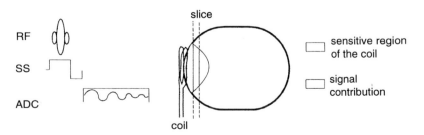

Figure 8.9. Schematic of the DRESS technique.

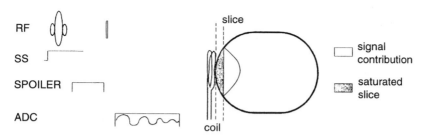

Figure 8.10. Schematic of the FROGS technique.

thogonal planes, to prepare the magnetization of the region of interest. The sequence is repeated eight times with various combinations of 180° excitations to coherently add signal from the region lying in the intersection of the selected slices. Although in practice three gradients are used to select a cubical region, we shall consider the simpler case of the two-dimensional ISIS.

Consider the effect of introducing a preinversion RF pulse (180°) in an FID sequence as shown in Figure 8.11. If the time elapsed between the 180 and 90° pulses is negligible in comparison to the relaxation time T1 of the spins, the effect will be the same as that of a 270° RF pulse. The signal detected from such an excitation (180, 90) will be opposite in phase, compared to one from a simple 90° excitation. The relation of the excitation scheme to the phase of the received signal is apparent from Figure 8.11.

If the two FIDs are signal averaged with the same receiver phase, complete cancellation will occur. If, however, the receiver phase is alternated, the two signals will add coherently. The 2D-ISIS sequence is an extrapolation of this exercise, as further described below.

Consider a planar sample as in Figure 8.12, the plane of the sample being the *xy* plane. The ISIS pulse sequence cycle consists of four separate acquisitions, varying in the specifics of the slice preinversions, as shown on the left of the figure. The four FIDs

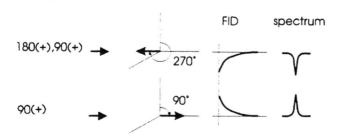

Figure 8.11. The effect of a preinversion RF pulse on the phase of the received signal.

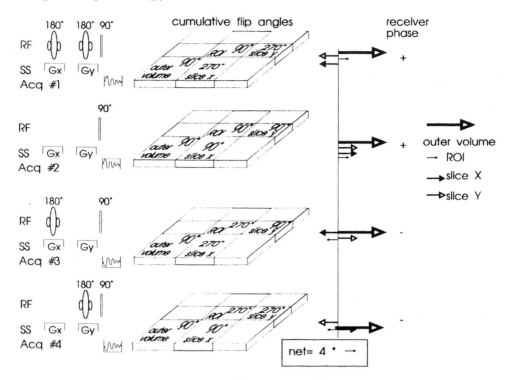

Figure 8.12. A two-dimensional ISIS sequence.

are then summed according to the prescribed receiver phase. The sample may be partitioned into four regions for the purpose of signal analysis. The 180° RF–G_x inversion will affect a slice region (labeled slice x); the 180° RF–G_y inversion will affect an orthogonal slice region (labeled slice y). The intersection of the two slices is the region of interest (labeled ROI). The rest of the sample region is labeled outer volume. The cumulative flip angles for each region are labeled in the midsection of the figure for each of the four acquisitions. The vectors corresponding to each region are shown on the right of the figure. At the end of each cycle, signals from acquisitions 1, 2 are added and those from acquisitions 3, 4 are subtracted. Upon summation of signals for each region (negate the sign when receiver phase is negative), it is seen that the signals from all the regions except the ROI will cancel.

One of the primary advantages of using this method is that the FID of the ROI is acquired immediately after the 90° pulse. This timing prevents signal losses due to T2 relaxation and is thus suitable for phosphorus spectroscopy. The ISIS method can suffer from dynamic range problems if the ROI is relatively small compared to the whole sample. The outer volume can be minimized by using a surface coil for signal reception.

Stimulated Echo Acquisition Mode (STEAM)

Chapter 1 described the formation of a Hahn spin echo as a result of applying a 90°, 180° RF pulse pair. The stimulated echo acquisition mode (STEAM) technique is based on the stimulated echo pulse sequence. A stimulated echo is produced when the sample experiences three 90° radio frequency pulses in succession. In fact, the application of three RF pulses will generate five echoes, one being the spin echo and an other the stimulated echo. The maximum amplitude of the stimulated echo is obtained when 90° pulses are used. If the 90° RF pulses are combined with appropriate slice selection gradients in one or more directions, a cubical volume of the sample that experiences the three RF excitations can be selected. This technique was first proposed by Frahm et al. as a means of generating localized proton spectra. The time delays between the pulses are shown in Figure 8.13. The period between the first and second RF pulses corresponds to half the echo time (TE). The period between the second and third RF pulses corresponds to the mixing time (TM). The period between the third RF pulse and the center of the echo is also equal to half the echo time.

The chief disadvantage of this method is that only half the spin magnetization contributes to echo formation. Furthermore, the stimulated echo experiences both T1 and T2 decay. The T2 decay occurs during the echo times: that is, between the first and second RF pulses and after the third RF pulse. T1 decay occurs during the mixing period TM. Typical times for TE and TM are 30 and 50 ms, respectively. To selectively detect the stimulated echo, the spin echoes and FIDs from one or more of the slice selections are carefully dephased while the stimulated echo signal is preserved. This is accomplished by proper design of slice selection gradient waveforms, as shown in Figure 8.13. Along

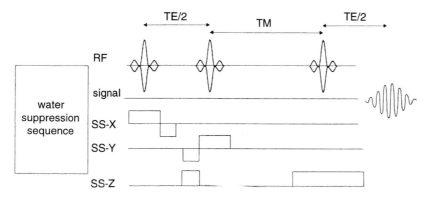

Figure 8.13. Pulse sequence for a water-suppressed STEAM experiment.

each axis, the slice-selected signal is rephased using the proper gradient pulse during the entire TE/2 + TM + TE/2 period. The gradient pulses after the second RF pulse prevent the formation of spin echoes. The gradient pulses placed after the third RF pulse provide rephasing for the stimulated echo signal as well as crushers for the FID signal. Because of the T2 losses, the STEAM technique is most suitable for localized proton spectroscopy, since phosphorus metabolites possess short T2s.

One of the prerequisites for proton spectroscopy is presaturation of the water resonance. The water resonance at 4.76 ppm is approximately 10^4 times stronger than the other metabolites. A proton spectrum without suppression of the water resonance cannot be used to detect weaker metabolites because of the finite dynamic range of the signal digitizer. A presaturation pulse sequence for water suppression is generally appended to the beginning of the STEAM sequence, as shown in the pulse sequence diagrams.

The main advantage of the STEAM method is that the spectrum from an ROI can be recorded in a single scan. Unlike ISIS, STEAM is not prone to subtraction errors. Furthermore, the volume selected can be readily imaged by simple modification of the sequence, and the coordinates of the ROI can be arbitrarily varied by appropriate design of the RF pulses.

Phase-Encode-Based Techniques

The alternate approach to slice selection is to use gradient pulses for the phase encoding of data, just as in MR imaging. The method may be implemented in one or more directions to achieve spatial resolution. This spectroscopy technique is referred to as chemical shift imaging (CSI). The term CSI has also been applied to an unrelated problem of selectively recording fat or water images. All references to CSI in this chapter pertain to the spectroscopic technique. A subcategory of CSI known as spectroscopic imaging (SI) has also been reported. The SI method differs from CSI only in the presentation of collected data.

Chemical shift imaging provides a way to obtain metabolite maps over the entire volume of a sample without resorting to slice selection gradients. Figure 8.14 shows the pulse sequence for a typical one-dimensional CSI sequence. Immediately following a nonselective RF pulse, a phase-encode gradient is turned on, whereupon the FID signal is recorded (without the use of a readout gradient pulse). This sequence is repeated as the gradient pulse is stepped through a set of values. The criteria used for the phase encoding are the same ones used in conventional MRI and depend on the desired field of view and spatial resolution. A

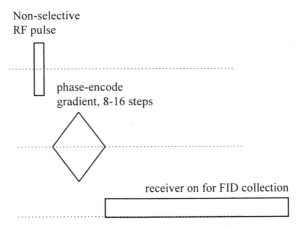

Figure 8.14. Pulse sequence for 1D-CSI ^{31}P spectroscopy.

2D data set generated in this example is processed by 2D Fourier transform algorithm as in conventional spin-echo imaging. The data set obtained corresponds to a series of spectra. These spectra originate from a series of slices along the direction of the phasing code gradient. If phase encoding is performed along two different directions using two different gradient pulses, a 3D data set will be obtained, which in turn can be used to resolve spectral information along two directions. The advantage of using this technique is that no slice selection artifacts are present in the data. Also, T2 losses can be minimized by collecting the FID signal. There are a few disadvantages, however. The use of phasing code gradients can lead to Gibbs artifacts that become manifest as blurring of the localized regions. The delay period introduced between the RF pulse and the beginning of data acquisition leads to excessive chemical shift dependent phase shifts. Although compensating for these phase shifts by postprocessing is difficult, the overall simplicity of the CSI technique has gained it wide acceptance.

The spectroscopic imaging (SI) is related to CSI technique in that phase-encode gradients in one or more directions are utilized to localize the information. Typically, whole-volume data (e.g., from the brain) are collected using a 3D CSI pulse sequence. The 3D FT-processed data then are presented as a set of low resolution images corresponding to each spectral resonance. For phosphorus spectroscopic imaging, an FID sequence is used. For proton spectroscopic imaging a water-suppressed, spin-echo pulse sequence is used. The primary advantage of this technique is that the ROI does not have to be determined before the study is begun. However, acquisition of a spectroscopic imaging data set can be time-consuming.

Selected Clinical Applications

We have described a number of pulse sequence techniques that allow acquisition of volume-selective spectra. Each sequence, with its inherent set of advantages and disadvantages, has been found to be useful for certain specific applications. Let us now examine some common examples of spectroscopic examinations.

Muscle Spectroscopy

Normal muscle is abundant in high energy metabolites such as ATP and phosphocreatine (PCr) and is thus amenable to phosphorus spectroscopy. Moreover, the calf and forearm muscles are relatively superficial and are accessible by means of surface coils. Appropriate exercise protocols can be used to monitor the status of aerobic and anaerobic metabolism. The changes in in-

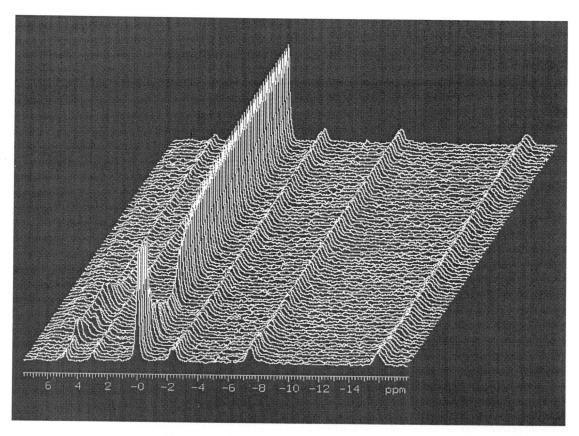

Figure 8.15. Changes in ^{31}P spectra of muscle during exercise. Courtesy of Dr. Alan Roth.

tensities of resonances and the pH (derived from the chemical shift of P_i) are monitored before, during, and after the exercise regimen. A number of metabolic disorders have been examined by means of phosphorus spectroscopy. Some examples are McArdle's syndrome, glycogen storage disease, and Duchenne's muscular dystrophy.

Figure 8.15 shows a set of spectra recorded by means of a surface coil during a period of calf muscle (gastrocnemius) exercise.

After the onset of exercise, the intensity of the P_i resonance increases and that of PCr decreases. During this process, the pH of tissue decreases, as evidenced by the shift to right of P_i peak. After cessation of exercise, immediate recovery of the PCr is noted, concurrent with fall of P_i. The pH, however, is slow to recover.

Brain Spectroscopy

Several disease conditions, such as dementia and epileptic seizures, do not always manifest themselves in routine MRI and are thus good candidates for spectroscopic examination. Spectroscopy has also been proposed as a means of predicting tumor treatment response, and for the characterization of radiation necrosis. Most spectroscopic brain examinations performed to date involve the use of single-voxel methods (ISIS or STEAM) or the SI technique. Figure 8.16 presents a proton spectrum recorded from a patient with a history of seizures. Figure 8.16a shows a voxel grid from which the spectra are recorded. A spectrum from voxels representing a normal region appear in Figure 8.16b. A spectrum from the abnormal region had lower relative amounts of NAA, the neuronal marker, than were present in healthy tissue.

Liver Spectroscopy

Surface coil spectroscopy is used in acquiring phosphorus spectra from liver. Several methods have been reported for liver studies, including FROGS, DRESS, ISIS, and CSI. Figure 8.17 is an example of a 1D CSI data set from a normal subject, using a 10 cm surface coil. Because of paramagnetic components present in the liver (note relative to short T1 of liver tissue), the resonance lines are generally broader than those for muscle or brain tissue. The resonance corresponding to the external reference is observed in the first two spectra. Progressing further into the stack, spectra from outlying muscle appear. The rather strong

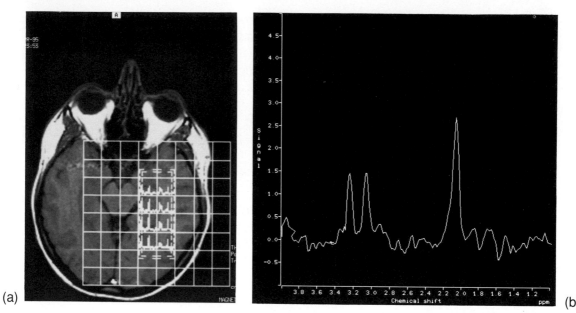

(a)

(b)

Figure 8.16. A water-suppressed proton spectrum acquired by means of the two-dimensional spectroscopic imaging pulse sequence, (a) Graphic representation of voxel positioning. (b) Proton spectrum from normal region of the temporal lobe of an epilectic patient.

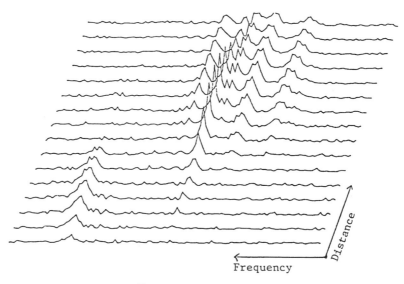

Figure 8.17. Localized ^{31}P spectra obtained from 1D-CSI; each spectrum represents a 5 mm slab of liver tissue. Forefront of figure represents area closest to surface coil. In the first few spectra, the far left peak is a signal from a reference vial on the surface of the subject's body. (Courtesy of K. J. Myers.)

PCr peak from muscle extends deep into the spectral stack as a consequence of Gibbs ringing artifact. Liver spectra are devoid of the PCr resonance.

The few examples presented above serve only to illustrate the breadth of this subject and are by no means comprehensive. Although NMR spectroscopy holds much promise for the noninvasive evaluation of metabolism, only a few applications have made their way into the clinical setting. Nonetheless, spectroscopic imaging of metabolites will continue to be an active area of research in the near future.

Additional Reading

Frahm J, Michaelis T, Merbolt KD et al. Localized NMR spectroscopy in vivo: Progress and problems. *NMR Biomed* 2, 188–195 (1988).

Ross B, Michaelis T. Clinical applications of magnetic resonance spectroscopy. *Magn Resonance Q* 10(4), 191 (1994).

Appendix

k-Space Formalism

Fourier Space or *k*-Space

An alternate way to understand MRI acquisition schemes is through the concept of Fourier space, or *k*-space. Although the concept of Fourier space is not intuitively easy to understand, it provides a unified view of all data acquisition schemes used in imaging. Some pulse sequence methods, such as echo-planar imaging, are best understood by way of the concept of Fourier space. The basic premise of the *k*-space formalism is that any image can be entirely described by its content in spatial frequencies: that is, how information varies across the image. Thus, for any image there exists a complementary image containing the spatial frequencies. Although the term "spatial frequencies" appears unintuitive, it can be understood by examining the sound waveform analogy. Any sound waveform can be decomposed into a sum of elementary frequencies having various amplitudes and phases. One can reconstruct the waveform by appropriate combination of the component frequencies.

Let us examine further the concept of spatial frequency as it pertains to an image. Since images have two dimensions, spatial frequencies must be separated in perpendicular directions, say x and y. A spatial frequency may be seen as the number of times the information in the image changes per unit length of the image. For instance, let us consider an "infinite" image made of points spaced every inch in the x direction and every 2 inches in the y direction (Figure A.1). Therefore, the spatial frequency along x is 1 per inch and the spatial frequency along y is 0.5 per inch. One may exactly reconstruct the actual image from knowledge of these spatial frequencies.

A more complicated image would require more than two spatial frequencies, but the principles remain the same. And conversely, the actual image can be exactly reconstructed from knowledge of the spatial frequency components. The mathematical operation that is used to go from the Fourier space to

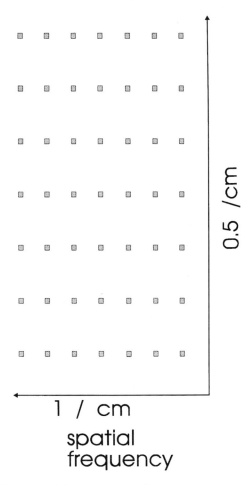

Figure A.1. The spatial frequencies of an image comprising a matrix of dots.

the actual space or vice versa is called **Fourier transformation** (Figure A.2). These frequencies are usually called *kx* and *ky*, with the result that the Fourier space is also called *k*-space. In this space, low frequencies correspond to slow variations across the image and therefore contain information about contrast. High spatial frequencies correspond to rapid variations in the image and encode details. The resolution in the image is given by the highest spatial frequencies that may be found in the image.

The Fourier space has certain interesting features that are also found in holography, which is based on Fourier analysis. For instance, a given point in the Fourier space does not correspond to a given point in the actual image. A point in the Fourier space is associated with a given set of two spatial frequencies, one along *x* and the other along *y*. These frequencies contribute to the entire image. Fourier imaging and Fourier transformation are used in many disciplines of physics and engineering. With MRI,

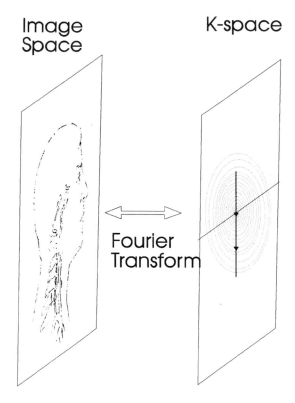

Figure A.2. The one-to-one correspondence between image space and *k*-space.

the link between Fourier space and images is direct, since data are collected in the computer memory in terms of spatial frequencies.

Phase Encoding

The *k*-space image is directly connected to the MRI image by the Fourier transform operation. As described in Chapter 2, the phase-encode technique provides an elegant way to encode the position of spins by virtue of their phase frequencies. The *k*-space formalism described below provides an alternate understanding of the process of phase encoding.

Using a constant gradient G_x, the precession frequency at location x is:

$$\nu(G_x, x) = gG_x x \qquad (A.1)$$

(The relation to equation 2.3 will be noted; equation A.1, however, refers to the rotating frame, with the result that the static field component is excluded.)

If G_x is applied during a given time interval t, spins will have precessed at an angle Ø determined by:

$$\phi = v(G_x, x)t = gG_x tx \qquad (A.2)$$

Since Ø must be between 0 and π radians, it appears that the phase varies cyclically along x axis ($gG_x t$) per unit length. The associated spatial frequency is thus

$$k_x = gG_x t \qquad (A.3)$$

Similarly, for a gradient G_y applied in the y direction, the corresponding spatial frequency along y axis would be:

$$k_y = gG_y t \qquad (A.4)$$

Hence, the spatial frequencies are proportional to the gradient amplitude and the duration of the gradient used to phase-encode spins. In as much as gradients may vary in time, spatial frequencies are more exactly defined as the integral over time of the gradient pulse shape (i.e., the area under the gradient pulses).

Basically, the k-space or Fourier space may be represented by two axes, k_x and k_y. For technological reasons, sampling of k-space must be discrete. An MRI acquisition may thus be seen as a series of data collections that will provide the amplitude and the phase of a given number of spatial frequencies. When the amplitude and the phase of those selected spatial frequencies are known, it is necessary to "reconstruct" the image by means of a Fourier transformation in both x and y directions.

The number and the pattern of spatial frequencies needed for the generation of an image depends on the features present (e.g., image resolution, field of view). The size of the k-space—that is, the highest spatial frequency that will be analyzed—determines the size of the smallest structure that can be seen in the image (pixel) (i.e., the image resolution). The pixel size p is therefore:

$$p_{x,y} = \frac{1}{k_{xy,max}} \qquad (A.5)$$

Since the maximum value achievable for k directly depends on the maximum gradient intensity available (equations A.3, A.4), image resolution is limited by gradient hardware. One may also increase the duration of the gradient, if this is not prevented by sequence design and signal-to-noise ratio limitations. The smallest step in Fourier space sampling or the distance between consecutive points, assuming all points are regularly spaced, determines the lowest spatial frequency that can be recognized. This frequency corresponds to the longest that can be seen in the image (i.e., to the field of view). Thus along the x and y directions, FOV$_{x,y}$ is

$$\text{FOV}_{x,y} = \frac{1}{k_{xy,\min}} \tag{A.6}$$

The number $n_{x,y}$ of k-space points to analyze in either direction x or y is therefore:

$$n_{x,y} = \frac{k_{xy,\max}}{k_{xy,\min}} = \frac{\text{FOV}_{x,y}}{P_{x,y}} \tag{A.7}$$

Thus $n_{x,y}$ is also the number of pixels in the actual image. Therefore, one must obtain information on as many points in the k-space as there are pixels in the actual image. Remember, however, that a point in the k-space does not correspond to a pixel in the actual image but is linked to the whole image.

Classical 2DFT Imaging

We now see how the concept of Fourier space applies to conventional spin-echo imaging. In conventional spin-echo imaging, spatial encoding is obtained through frequency and phase encoding as described in Chapter 2. During the pulse sequence, the data points are recorded during the readout period, and data acquisition is repeated for successive values of the phase-encode gradient. These data points, which are acquired sequentially, form the k-space image. This section describes the congruence of the data points to that of the k-space.

At the beginning of the pulse sequence, the spatial frequency is 0 in both x and y directions, corresponding to the center of the k-space (point A in Figure A.3). Typically, a gradient pulse is applied in the first half of the spin-echo sequence on the so-called readout axis. Let us call this axis x. The amplitude and duration of this pulse are fixed and determined, so that the corresponding k_x is $k_{x,\max}/2$, which is determined by image resolution. Simultaneously, a gradient pulse of variable amplitude is applied on the y axis for phase encoding, corresponding to a spatial frequency k_y. Therefore, after these two pulses we have traversed to position B in Figure A.3 (at the extremity of a line in k-space). As long as no other gradient pulse is applied either on x or y axis, the spatial frequencies remain the same. The effect of the 180° RF pulse is to invert the phase of the transverse magnetization, which in k-space results in symmetric reflection with respect to the center. We move now to position C in k-space. During the echo, a gradient pulse is applied (readout gradient). Signal inten-

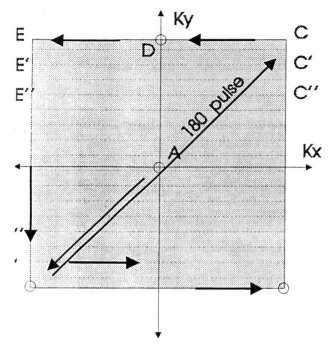

Figure A.3. The trajectory of data acquired during an spin-echo scan.

sity will be discretely sampled at regular intervals t. Each signal pickup will therefore be associated with a different spatial frequency along the x axis. Between two consecutive signal pickups, spatial frequency will have increased by $k_{x,min}$, which is determined by the field of view:

$$k_{x,min} = \gamma G_x t = \frac{1}{FOV_x} \tag{A.8}$$

In the k-space, the position of the data point being recorded moves from point C along the k_x direction, in steps of $k_{x,min}$, since k_y does not change. At the center of the echo, we have sampled $n_x/2$ points in k-space, putting us at point D, which must be at the center of the k_x line. For this purpose, we must satisfy the condition:

$$\frac{k_{x,max}}{2} = \frac{k_{x,min}n_x}{2} \tag{A.9}$$

which means that the area of the gradient pulse applied on the readout axis in the first period is identical to that of the readout gradient pulse from its start to the top of the echo. From the top of the echo, the signal is sampled symmetrically over $n_x/2$ points, up to the end of the k_x line (i.e., point E). Hence, the total duration of the readout gradient pulse is $n_x t$. On each side of the top of the echo, the signal drops according to T2*. One can see how the gradient pulse intensity, its duration, and the sampling rate are tied to the image resolution and the field of view. Shorter sampling times require stronger gradient pulses.

At this stage of the acquisition process, we have seen that the sampling of one echo signal for a few milliseconds provides data for a full line in *k*-space. To get data on all lines, we must repeat the whole process again, line after line. To change lines, the amplitude of the phase-encoding gradient is changed, whereupon another value of k_y is obtained, leading to another point B' in *k*-space. Basically, the phase-encoding gradient amplitude is changed, ensuring that the corresponding spatial frequencies will vary between $-k_{y,\max}/2$ and $+k_{y,\max}/2$ by n_y steps of $k_{y,\mathrm{mix}}$.

Dramatic reduction in scan time can be obtained by changing the algorithm used to scan the *k*-space. As seen above, conventional techniques as well as gradient-echo imaging techniques require the n_y lines of the *k*-space to be scanned individually. There are, however, other acquisition schemes in which several lines in the *k*-space are scanned during a single sequence cycle. This is the approach used in the pulse sequences based on RARE (rapid acquisition by refocused echo). Ultimately, the whole *k*-space may be scanned in a single cycle, as with echo-planar imaging (EPI).

Additional Reading

Twieg DB. The k-trajectory formulation of the imaging process with applications in analysis and synthesis of imaging methods. Med Phys 10:610 (1983).

Index